Pastoral Interventions

Pastoral Interventions

A Perceptive Ministry

Neville A. Kirkwood
D. Min., Dip. Theol., L.Th. MACC

Baal Hamon Publishers
Akure   London   New York

ISBN-10: 978-49565-4-3
ISBN-13: 978-978-49565-4-3

International Correspondence: Baal Hamon,
27 Old Gloucester Street, London,
WC1N 3AX,
England.

www.baalhamonpublishers.com
publishers@baalhamon.com

Contents

Dedication

To those ministering to those in need and the recipients of their Pastoral Care.

Foreword

Spirituality and Faith are two words lacking from the general vocabulary of the medical profession. Yet, these words are the fourth frontier for medicine complementing biological, psychological and sociological to help form the whole person.

Neville Kirkwood has known this for a long time and has been able to synthesise the importance of Faith and Spirituality into the dynamic of modern health care, not only in his writings but also by the very life he has, and is leading. He is the epitome of the person who not only can talk the talk but also does walk the walk. Not only is he the pastor's pastor but also the model of caring which should be emulated by all in the helping professions.

He has been prepared to go where few others have been. His work and thoughts about working with Muslim patients was not only timely but important for it brought us to understand and appreciate what was helpful in their medical care.

This book too is timely. Pastoral, or should I say Spiritual Care is being expanded as systems come to recognise that this is a dimension for far too long ignored. Strangely, we owe so much in health care to faith traditions and yet we seem to have written it out of the history of medicine.

This is a book which will enable not only those of faith, but also those who see themselves as humanists to recognise the importance of the pastoral presence in our Interventions, be they with patients, professionals or colleagues.

Pastoral Interventions is a model to enable the reader to reflect on situations and see possible solutions. The author knows that the solutions are not prescriptive but rather offer possibilities of processes that could be applied.

Religious language speaks about 'toiling in the vineyard of the Lord". Neville Kirkwood has given us something which enables that toiling to occur using many different instruments and tools. My tradition speaks about our task to make the world a better place than when we found it. In making it better, it should approach perfection enough that the messiah would not be necessary. Neville enables us to move to that place with both this book and his life.

Rabbi Jeffrey Cohen FRSA DD D.Min. BCC
Sydney Australia

Introduction

In Pastoral Ministry intervention meets men, women and children in many different states and conditions in which they may be floundering. The world to them may seem unrelenting, cold and indifferent to their plight. Well meaning friends and family may try to rescue them but in so doing add further confusion and make the situation worse.

A person who in the name of God or some helping organization comes to offer support in their hour of need must be aware of the pits into which they may fall in dealing with certain issues. Pastoral and community workers, if unaware, can make the same mistakes as the untrained friend or relative, compounding their disrupted life with further anguish. It is necessary that when pastoral care is offered it is going to bring the desired comfort, encouragement, perceptiveness and coping-strength to the one who is experiencing the distress.

Often such people are facing unprecedented circumstances in their lives. Their previously held frames of reference in handling life's situations under these new and different situations are inapplicable. They may be likened to babes lost in an unknown forest. Their cherished priorities do not fit what they are going through. Their intellectual assessments do not equate with the current happenings. Even, their cozy spiritual and theological conclusions do not compute with the new data. Thus, many of those, which are met on the daily round, have to make changes in their priorities and values. Re-adjustments to life outside their normal comfort zones have to be made.

In the following pages, a number of these situations, which unless managed rightly are able to cause mental, spiritual and physical harm, are looked at from the pastoral perspective. The issues dealt with are to be found in the community and in the congregation from time to time. Pastoral workers must be alert to them, be able to read the signs, and adequately assess their situation and act appropriately. On numerous occasions, I have been called to help those who have been further hurt or confused by well-meaning church members and pastoral visitors. Many such visitors think the reading of scripture and a prayer is the panacea for all occasions. Often, scripture and prayer are only effective after the hard and difficult spade work in confronting the problem had been done. In other cases, the person's faith has been so shattered that they need to feel some helpful and understanding support from the visitor before any God talk is able to be taken up.

Into such situations, the pastoral person must enter pre-armed by their own personal prayer for wisdom and guidance from God. To come to persons involved in the areas of need we will be looking to the indwelling Spirit of the living God who must be present providing the sensitivity and perceptiveness to deal with the person concerned. Without such support, it may be like picking off the scab from a wound and opening it to further infection. Jesus did not send his disciples out from Caesarea Philippi until he had sufficiently equipped them for the task.

In opening up the following possible pastoral situations it is to give you, the reader, a greater perception of the difficulties, confusion and anxiety the person is going through and with pastoral help may receive some healing of mind and spirit and be encouraged to face what lies ahead.

To understand what the person is likely to be thinking and feeling is one of the gifts of pastoral care. The purpose of this book is to provide information to assist in making you aware of the background of the condition so as to make the pastoral visit as smooth and as helpful as possible. It is not meant to be a definitive prescription of how to handle every patient as each person's condition, circumstances and reactions differ from others with similar diagnosis.

The God of the Torah, the Bible, the Koran, the Vedantas and the Yashna, all refer to a God whose spirit dwells in each human being and who is loved and considered precious in the eyes of the one supreme God. The pastoral person's role is to minister to these subjects of this eternal deity as if God himself were coming to their side whether in a hospital bed or elsewhere. The invitation is to you to explore and in some measure be practically informed about some of the challenges you may confront in your pastoral visiting.

CHAPTER 1

The Pastoral Person

The pastoral helper may be described as any person, man or woman, who sees another in need and moves to help. This help may take many forms from the provision of food, clothing, accommodation or comfort and assurance in severe illness, crisis or death. But not everyone who would help is equipped to meet these needs. It demands an understanding selfless person who has a heart that is not easily disconcerted or overwhelmed by the other's trauma. Special qualities and gifts are required of a pastoral person/carer.

Some people acquire a natural pastoral gift and are able to make a positive impact because of human experience, knowledge and perceptiveness. Someone ordained into Holy Orders may not necessarily be a good pastoral person. Their particular gifts may be in the areas of administration, preaching, teaching or program initiation. Neither are all members of the laity gifted for such sensitive situations.

The essential element of the pastoral helper is that they have a love for and an acceptance of people-whatever their background, beliefs or condition. They do not shrink from reaching out to one with HIV/Aids, a prostitute or a person grotesquely deformed or mutilated. Even those who have a pastoral gift will be much more effective after a serious commitment to ongoing study and training, in the areas of pastoral care, management of grief and loss and ministry skills. A caring heart without special training can be persuaded to take on responsibilities not properly theirs or given a false sense of their ability and achievements which may give them an unwarranted self-confidence for this ministry. The futility of such well intentioned caring can damage and break the enthusiasm of the person with the pastoral heart.

A person who desires a long term truly effective ministry will make serious efforts to enrich their God given pastoral gifts.

THE NATURE OF THE PASTORAL PERSON

The Heart of a Lover

A pastoral career has a heart that is open and responsive to all people, irrespective of class, color or creed. He or she will look upon people as Christ did and see the possibilities. They have a heart that can see the lovable in the unlovable and the potential in the dejected and depressed. It can see the gold in the murky silt of the stream of a person's tragic life. Beneath the filth of a disordered, debauched life he is gifted with the vision of a renewed, clean and focused life of possibility.

The pastoral person is a lover of humanity who recognizes and accepts the squalor and sadness, the unhappiness and the disheartening stress in the lives of others. Without feeling a need to be judgmental, they will sit where the other sits, identify with them and their problem, without any sense of aloofness, condescension, or superiority.

> *A pastoral career has a heart that is open and responsive to all people, irrespective of class, color or creed.*

Much of the missionary effort of the colonial period in third world countries did not achieve outstanding results. The missionaries aligned themselves with the colonial overlords who saw the indigenes as nothing more than poor ignorant pagans who needed lifting to some higher status. For a successful pastoral ministry, the first requirements are to: love the underprivileged, know them as friends, be their companion on the way and share their burden as they struggle to overcome their difficult circumstances.

To love with a pastoral heart is to show patience and perseverance. The response to care is seldom immediate. Trust comes as a result of many acts of faithfulness, kindness, understanding and a genuine concern that has been demonstrated over time. Sometimes we will seem to be making progress then there may be a sudden withdrawal of trust. This is often the case when dealing with a person with an alcohol, gambling or other problem. A true lover of people is not daunted by such relapses but persists. As we continue to encourage the needy one, confidence is being built up. It is a great source of personal encouragement to see any renewed effort to change and may well create a stronger determination by the needy one not to make the same mistake again. They may fail again but are usually more careful because they are ashamed that they let the carer down once again. The persistent love which the carer offers is often the key which opens the door to a normal, healthy, communicative life within society.

> *To love with a pastoral heart is to show patience and perseverance. The response to care is seldom immediate.*

An Open-minded Approach

We say, 'love is blind.' A lover usually concentrates on the loved one and very often has a closed mind or is not fully aware regarding matters of significance that are happening around him or her. A person with too conservative views on religious matters may find it difficult to appreciate or share another's view on issues of God and faith. Keeping an open and generous mind on matters of belief is important in gaining trust. But this caring love is not over-indulgent. Over-indulgent care means, the care is not in proportion to the need and does not allow the one being helped to lift themselves out of their situation.   Over-indulgence creates a dependence upon the carer which adds to the problem. The needy person does not receive the necessary challenge to develop the strength to stand alone.

Open-mindedness means that there is less danger of being engrossed and absorbed in the presenting problem. If the carer keeps an open mind, the problem we are addressing and the circumstances stay in perspective. Let us take the alcoholic again. It is easy to see that alcohol consumption is a real problem. Much time can be spent by talking about alcohol abuse, providing distractions and diversions to minimize the opportunities for drinking or providing a non-alcoholic environment. The caring person does not narrow the problem to the presenting issue e.g. alcoholism. The pastoral person sees that the alcoholic is often forced into alcoholism by trying to escape the pressures of other external or personal issues.

> *A person with too conservative views on religious matters may find it difficult to appreciate or share another's view on issues of God and faith.*

Such issues may include an inferiority complex rising from rejection, failure to achieve, a broken relationship, guilt over personal misconduct, denigration by others etc. These are issues which need to be addressed before you are able to be sure he is able enough to understand the issues and make the reform permanent. The open-minded pastoral worker is able to work on several core issues which need to be dealt with, either simultaneously or one at a time with a minor problem first, then proceeding to the more serious ones. Trust has to be built up gradually.

An open mind and experience in human problems enables the pastoral helper to remain calm and undisturbed by any new revelation in the process which has brought about the addiction. An open heart and calm mind offering love and acceptance, can often provide a way for the patient to find wholeness and peace.

The Practice of Perception.

Meeting a troubled person for the first time is like taking a hand in a game of poker. So much of the troubled one's life will be unknown to you. Aspects of his or her life will vary in quality and value. The other's cards are kept close to the chest and are not revealed until the carer makes the right move to encourage them to throw one or more of their cards onto the table.

Successful poker players are able to read the signs and reactions of the opposite player as they have their hand dealt, or take up a card. The pastoral helper too needs to be able to read the facial expressions and indicators that the person is showing whether they are pleased or otherwise at the latest move in the game.

When making a home visit, your entry into the home may reveal much to the observant pastoral visitor. If the house or room is neat and tidy, the person may be able to manage their household chores, has an able partner, or has a cleaning person to attend to those needs. It does not take long to decide which of these is the case. An ability to fend for themselves often is an indication of their mental, physical, emotional and in some cases their spiritual strengths or otherwise. If there are some positives in these areas, it is often wise to make some complimentary remarks. This is an important way in which you can lessen any feeling they may have that you will be critical or make unfair judgments. Some people may be apprehensive about a visit from a church pastoral visitor; apprehensive about any report going back to the church fellowship. Be acutely aware of this. Give them your assurance that if a report is made, they will share in it. Remember you are also being watched and assessed for your integrity.

If there is any known physical or medical condition for this visit, you may be able to make an assessment of the extent and seriousness of the condition as you observe their movements, their speech, their clarity of mind and their willingness to be open about it, or their efforts to avoid any reference to it.

Some people have a deep need to protect their privacy and maintain their independence. They will conceal their condition as far as possible. The acute observer can detect whether all their statements about themselves ring true. Their "I'm OK" may well be an indication that they don't want to talk to you about their problem; and that they don't really welcome your visit. By observing their body language you should quickly decide on the wisdom of making a shortened visit and whether a further visit would have any value. If there are signs of strong objections, it is important to try to keep the door open for a further visit by yourself or another helper if the circumstances change.

> *Some people have a deep need to protect their privacy and maintain their independence. They will conceal their condition as far as possible.*

Make your visit short if you note that the person is in pain, under heavy medication, is not able to concentrate on what is being said or even has difficulty in realizing who you are. Such circumstances only further stress the patient.

If the one being visited feels that their situation is grossly unfair and that they are not deserving of their situation, they may be angry toward God who allows it to happen. In such a situation, deal with it as directly as possible. In fact any suggestion that God knows best or that God understands may destroy your credibility as a pastoral visitor and in such cases to suggest a parting prayer or scripture reading would be offensive.

The wise pastoral person is trained to be aware of what to do or not do or say in order to develop friendly feelings and confidence in the unconditional support and integrity of the pastoral visitor.

Being Perceptive

A heart sensitive to the needs of the person you are visiting may be the most important quality you can bring to the situation. It will show you where to give comfort and assurance to the one crying out for relief and reassurance. Of course, some will be stoutly and hostilely opposed. The person being visited may have a chip on his or her shoulders about the church because of a previous unhappy experience. A sense of false pride over accepting help from others or the loss of independence and the admission of need is an embarrassment. The perceptive person also is careful not to aggravate such feelings. A sensitive person's comfort and assurance is able to touch the heart where it is wanted and needed.

Having a heart sensitive to others' needs, means that the motive for the visit is not self-achievement nor to report to the next church meeting of another success statistic. The person you are visiting has a particularly stressful situation which needs to be eased. The sensitive heart has developed the perceptive skills necessary to pick up each sign of extra concern, anxiety, stress or discomfort being experienced. Such discernment also includes an awareness of the willingness or otherwise of the troubled one to share what is going on in their life or body. Learning to be perceptive and sensitive in these situations will enable you to assess how far and how quickly the life and mental problems of the other may be open to you.

Having a heart sensitive to others' needs, means that the motive for the visit is not self-achievement nor to report . . .

When you visit a pastoral patient, he or she will be quick to assess your understanding of their problem and situation. Will any personal revelations be received appropriately and empathically? True sensitivity and perceptiveness are able to reach the heart and encourage a response in the patient to produce the comfort and assurance that the pastoral person is seeking to achieve. A sensitive person will not make any observation or criticism until obstructions to positive communication and help have been cleared away. The pastoral person should not assume to probe into the personal concerns of the other. Wait until that right is given.

Subtle and Persistent

Subtle and persistent are terms which appear contradictory to what we have just said about sensitivity. Subtle may mean wiry, crafty, clever or insidious. These are not the meaning in this context. The subtle approach of the pastoral person may be said to involve a discriminating use of opportunities – a tactful approach would or will not give offence or cause undue anxiety.

To be persistent may conjure up the picture of a terrier with a rag doll; not satisfied until it has torn it to pieces in the quickest possible time. It can also mean being naggingly insistent in spite of obvious opposition. Persistence in these two interpretations involves a sense of continuing in a manner which is undesirable, aggravating and objectionable. This is not the way an experienced pastoral helper should respond when the acceptance is less than cordial. A persistent pastoral visitor is one who is not easily offended or abandons a person where the visit is less than warm. The pastoral person recognizes that he or she may not be welcome but does not display any hurt or feeling of slight and thus lessen the potential for good in this visit. Instead the tactful, persistent approach is likely to allow for further visits until the genuine interest and care of the visitor can be perceived and accepted.

The pastoral person will offer friendliness and acceptance of the person as a person in spite of the lack of reciprocal cordiality being shown. Avoid any offence by ignoring any rebuff and remain warm and caring on each visit.

I recall a couple of left-wing agitators openly stirring up hostility among the residents of a Christian mission working amongst a deprived, indigenous group. The workers at the mission did not openly oppose them and openly greeted them with hospitable friendliness. The mission conducted the only medical facility for a hundred miles and it so happened that one of these agitators took seriously ill and was forced to turn up on the mission doorstep seeking medical help. She received the best of care and recovered without complications. The remark she made to the medical staff was, "You will win us by love yet." The mission staff actually saved that woman's life. Such is the nature of subtle persistence. The lines of communication are kept open even when withdrawal may seem the right course.

When these valuable skills are cultivated and practiced by the pastoral person even the most persistent opposition can be broken down and even the hardest of hearts become amenable under this treatment. These are magical keys to open an awareness to penetrate to the core of hurting human hearts. Love, openheartedness, observation, sensitivity, and tact combined can bring even to the unwilling ones comfort, assurance, ease of mind and a calm spirit.

THE TASK OF THE PASTORAL PERSON.

Try to avoid planning all aspects of your next visit unless and until you can be sure you know him or her sufficiently to assess their attitude and what they require of you.   Such an approach most likely will be mechanical and forced. It does not take into account that the mood of the one visited may be different from the previous visit because of what may have happened in the interim of which you are unaware. One of the positives of seeing the same hospital patient daily is that the chaplain is able to observe the person in different states of mind. You cannot necessarily expect to see the same patient feeling the same the next day. The patient or the one visited has to be reassessed on each visit. The approach to the same person may vary from visit to visit. If the visit is to be of positive value, it must attend to the needs of the day.

The pastoral visitor's task on any visit may be able to:
  ➢ Awaken to reality
  ➢ Encourage a vision of purpose and usefulness
  ➢ Liberate from a sense of guilt
  ➢ Ease the pain of grief
  ➢ Offer support when all seems hopeless
  ➢ Broaden the picture to include others.
  ➢ Soften the severity of the situation
  ➢ Strengthen the mind and body for action.
  ➢ Lift from the slough of despondency

Awaken to Reality

Many people who are passing through troubled waters whether it is illness, bereavement, financial hardship, unemployment and failure to achieve goals, severe disappointment, a relationship breakdown or other hurt will require pastoral support. Their current problem fills their mind and blocks out normal mental activity. It is producing anxiety, stress and almost certainly affecting their work colleagues, family members and others. They are unable to concentrate and give the required effort to their work and other duties. They are spending time in anguish over the matter magnifying in their mind the painfulness and the disorder the issue is having upon their lives.

The concentration of mental resources used to grapple with the problem, may well be out of proportion to actual situation. The internal brooding usually focuses upon the negative factors. The more negative scores they mark up the gloomier and more pessimistic the situation appears. The door is open to depression even may revisit other past unhappy situations and so displace all peace and rational thinking.

When the pastoral visitor arrives, he or she may be seen as one who may well provide a sympathetic ear. It may not be a helpful situation if the visitor's presence is seen merely as one from whom to gain sympathy, to secure answers and favors. If the pastoral helper does not see this, it can lead into deeper feelings of helplessness even hopelessness. Many in these circumstances are unable to separate the reality of the situation from the distortions they have built up. It is possible their outpourings to the visitor only add more somber colors to the picture in their mind. Of course the possibility of being manipulated must always be considered particularly in the early stages of the relationship.

On the other hand, it may be therapeutic to unburden anxieties to a pastoral carer. It brings the problem(s) out into the open so that the situation may be viewed from a more objective aspect that the visitor is able to open out. This should aim for the person to sort out a solution for themselves rather than telling them or advising what they should do.

Such reflective listening and response helps to provide a balanced approach and importantly reestablish self-confidence and self-esteem.

The pastoral person's responsibility is to try and provide some element of reality. This can only be done bit by bit in a gentle and quiet manner. Distortion and fabrications must be taken apart caringly to allow the true scene to be brought more into perspective; to awaken the mind to reality and the positive and encouraging possibilities available to them.

Encourage a Vision of Usefulness.
Having been able to lessen the emotionally charged tension and anxiety in the other, the pastoral carer is able to start to encourage the building of a vision of usefulness. The visitor can now rationally discuss ways in which they can reassume a useful role in society, even if there is some impairment. If he or she has been convinced of this, then much has been achieved. The reappraisement of their condition will be more balanced and they are likely to be more cheerful among family, friends and colleagues.

Without some sense of being able to make some useful contribution in life, the depression and pessimism is likely to become pathological with strong, negative repercussions for relationships with kin, colleagues and close friends. Nobody wants to be in the company of someone who has a perpetual long face along with much doom and gloom conversational patter.

As a person, Simpson was a well regarded man who was happily married with a wife of twenty-five years. They had no children. Sybil, his wife, was diagnosed with cancer with well advanced secondaries into the kidney and liver. Within five weeks of exploratory surgery which proved the cancer was inoperable she had died. Naturally, Simpson was shocked, dumbfounded. His grief was agonizing. Many caring visitors came to visit him but he was inconsolable. He withdrew from social contact, even his church, and became virtually a recluse. He became so inefficient at work that after being patient for several months his employer had to dismiss him. In one way Simpson was relieved, because he no longer had to associate with those at his work place. He withdrew further into himself.

George was the one person from his church who continued to visit him periodically. Sybil has been involved with "Meal on Wheels" delivering meals two days a week to shut–ins and the incapacitated elderly. She was also a volunteer involved in helping out at the Church's Opportunity Shop which sold second-hand clothing, furniture, household accessories etc.

George on his visits would sometimes mention what a valuable asset Sybil was and spoke warmly of how much she was missed by the Meals on Wheels team. He sometimes recalled just how much pleasure Sybil gave to those she visited and to those who came to the Opportunity Shop. Simpson's face would lighten up at these tributes to his wife's charm and outgoing nature.

After a few weeks, of returning to such themes George pointed out that there was a shortage of volunteers for both delivering Meals on Wheels and the Op Shop. He said that he thought Sybil would be unhappy with the situation. After a time, he accepted George's point of view and then it became easier for George to suggest that he could honor Sybil's memory by continuing in these roles which gave her such a sense of fulfillment.

It took time before the vision became a reality. Simpson became a "Meal on Wheels" driver and earned their appreciation and approval. Simpson's smile began to come back. He soon after became an Op. Shop volunteer sorting and pricing the goods, and his happy smile came back. His continuing efficiency gained him promotion to Receiving Room Supervisor. It was another twelve months before he was fully integrated back into the life of the church, other social activities and more importantly into full time employment. George the pastoral person brought Simpson back from serious depression into a state in which he could see himself as again useful in the world. George's skills and sensitivity to Simpson's condition enabled him to resume a restored productive place in his society.

Liberates From a Sense of Guilt.

Perplexing and dispiriting problems affect most people many times over a life span. Whether you are the visitor or the visited, when you face a pressing stressful episode there will be times of short or longer duration when you may have regrets over some things you have said or done. You may feel that the situation could have been made easier or even avoided if you had handled the situation differently. Things said or done are not easily retractable or the hurt or damage repaired. These regrets will recur to upset us and disturb the ability to concentrate on other and perhaps more important matters. They may make sleep restless and elusive.

Regret is a softer word for guilt for that is what it really is. It is a persistent feeling of guilt over something that has happened in the past. It may have involved something involving the family or with wider social implications relating to a single person, a group or a larger number of people. Some regrets can keep coming back for decades. It may have been something that has been kept closeted since childhood. It may have been done in childhood innocence or with childhood maliciousness. It may have hurt some other child or a person to a greater or lesser degree. In other circumstances, that guilt may be due to an oversensitive nature. The harm done may be perceived as greater than it really was. It might have been purely accidental without any opportunity for personal control. Guilt may recur as a feeling of dissatisfaction or irritation but depending upon its nature, work or act may torment disturbing our days and even our sleep.

Forgiveness does not imply that the episode can be forgotten nor by forgiveness are we condoning what was done.

Stuart broke a piece of Royal Doulton china, a precious family heirloom, when he was still at primary school. He picked up the pieces and hid them. It caused a furor in the household without anyone admitting to knowledge of what happened. The guilt was twofold. First there was guilt over the breakage; secondly the lies accompanying the cover up.

That incident was relived frequently until middle age when a caring pastoral person picked up the problem. It may seem a trivial event but at that time in the life of a very sensitive boy who had a fear of displeasing God, he could not shake the impression from his subconscious.

More seriously, a teenage prank resulted in a fatal vehicle accident, the cause of which was unresolved by the police or the coroner's inquiry. The instigator of the disaster was so wracked with secret guilt that he failed to finish his schooling, and was unable to settle into any regular employment. He showed signs of severe psychological problems and an inability to relate to others. During one of his hospital admissions, for the first time in just over 20 years, he told his story to the chaplain, who spoke with the family and the psychotherapist. Between them they were able to reassure him of an understanding God who forgives. The known survivor of the accident who lived in the same suburb was contacted. She had made a new and successful life and had long since, within herself, forgiven the one who caused the accident and was now able to do it face to face. The release from the torment of his guilt enabled him to readjust his life to include enrollment in a mature aged trade course and in time became an effective tradesman.

> *A pastoral person needs to be aware of the role guilt plays in the lives of many that he or she will visit.*

A pastoral person needs to be aware of the role guilt plays in the lives of many that he or she will visit. If you, as a visitor, have some prior knowledge or even a hint dropped in the conversation that guilt may be a causal factor of his inner turmoil, be wise, be sensitive, be observant and seek to find the truth in what is told to you.

A sense of guilt can only be picked up by listening to the story and making your own assessment of his or her actual role in the incident. Absence from the situation may be the cause of the guilt. They were not present to dampen down the event and so minimize the damage. By talking out the reasons for the guilt assumption, there can be a proper assessment of the problem and the best way to deal with the guilt question. In some cases, guilt may require him or her to seek forgiveness. True forgiveness begins with a need for self-forgiveness, which can only come from sincere repentance and a resolve to make amends and not repeat the offence. The pastoral person who can guide his patient into such forgiveness frees the troubled one from guilt and gives him, or her, a new sense of freedom.

Forgiveness does not imply that the episode can be forgotten nor by forgiveness are we condoning what was done. True forgiveness results in the event no longer influencing and disturbing our lives. It has been moved to the outer fringes of our concerns. As with any wound, scars often remain but do not adversely affect our ongoing lives. The lesson has been learned. When a small child drags a hot saucepan from the stove and is scalded the scars remain but the child is unlikely to repeat the mistake. Pastoral care is able to assist in releasing the continuing harmful impact of guilt. Such liberation may restore peace to a troubled mind, may heal broken relationships and allow the person to move forward.

Eases the Pain of Grief

Pastoral care often involves dealing with people who have been plunged into the depths of grief. They are struggling to rise above the severity of the pain. The real dimensions of the loss will depend upon the nature of the relationship between the mourner and the person or thing lost. Each person has their own measure of strength or ability to cope with loss. One may quickly adjust and make new attachments or find a replacement to cope with the loss. Another may lose spirit or motivation to rise up, to adjust and make a new start.

One of the aspects of grief, a pastoral person must remember is that any loss is an absence of the familiar. To move residence can build up as much grief in some as the death of a family member. This absence and loss has to be dealt with. It may be with silence without chatter to allow the reality of the loss to be absorbed. Talking about the pros and cons of the loss or just the continuous repetition of events and persons associated with the lost person or object are the ways some may seek to cope with their loss.

Whatever the case, the presence of a gifted pastoral person can ease the pain of grief. Silence or absence is one of the stark realities of a death in a family. Those who need to be silent to work through their loss often appreciate the presence of someone who will just sit. This is not only supportive but helps to lessen the feeling of loneliness. The silent presence of one just holding your hand can be of immense comfort.

Grief may involve aspects of the patient's life, that require help and healing but with which the untrained pastoral person cannot be expected to deal. Many complex issues are stirred up by a significant loss, such as guilt over unfinished business, the inability to say a proper goodbye, fears of the inability to manage affairs without the deceased, incompetence to continue or complete work and commitments left unfinished.

The pastoral person's role may be simply be that of a presence to give assurance that the one grieving will not have to face the future without God or the assistance of God's people. The sensitive and informed carer may indicate non-specific sources and help in some cases.

Many an hour has been spent saying and doing little with a person deep in grief to hear them say after their grief has been resolved, *"I don't know how I'd have coped without you being there for me."* Perhaps that may be all God or the person expected of you as a pastoral person in that situation.

The criteria for effective pastoral care in the time of grief are that it is appropriate to the person's situation and temperament and that the presence of the pastoral person eases the grief.

Supports When All Seems Hopeless

When a person's world has been turned upside down, the confusion makes it difficult to clearly see or get things in perspective. The future may seem bleak and hopeless. Their usual optimism and capacity to believe that better times will come cannot be entertained. The confidence that life is worthwhile disappears. A person in such a state of mind may well be your next patient.

Your care may rescue such a person from utter despair or suicide. Ben had been laid off by his employer as a result of downsizing and cost cutting in a search for ways to increase profits for the shareholders. Ben and Marilyn had four children, two going to secondary school and two still in primary classes. Like most young families they had a large mortgage on their home in a middle class suburb. House repayments devoured much of their monthly check. The threat of the house being auctioned over their heads and the move to a less affluent area where rents were cheaper was confusing and frightening. The future looked bleak and the parents were almost sick with worry. There seemed no way out; their future happiness and well being was in real peril.

> *When a person's world has been turned upside down, the confusion makes it difficult to clearly see or get things in perspective.*

John, a pastoral person, was asked by the school chaplain, to visit Ben and Marilyn. John felt for the family as he listened to their story. He could imagine himself in their position.

As John listened, he realized the underlying note of panic. He did pray from his heart for this couple. He promised to see what he could do. Ben and Marilyn thought, "Talk's cheap. What can he do?" that might be helpful.

Ben had worked for a building company and developer and was a very practical person with a trade certificate. Marilyn had trained as a teacher and was a skilled computer person who believed a stay at home mum was best for their children. The church had many people who needed home renovations and maintenance. There were many older members in the community who lacked computer skills and wanted to learn.

Through the active help and support of the church members, Ben received some daily work on house repairs and then advanced to larger renovations. Soon he registered himself as a business. The church organized a computer school on church premises for senior citizens. Church members donated computers that they no longer used because of updating. By charging a tuition fee Marilyn was also able to meet some of the family's expenses. By John's sensitive understanding and the church's response, this couple was able to continue life in their own home, in the same neighborhood, with the same church fellowship and Marilyn was still able to be home for the children after school.

Looking beyond the existing situation, the pastoral person and the church were able to transform a hopeless situation into even more fruitful and spiritually rewarding one. A pastoral carer, using the Christian love and support of the church, may turn seemingly hopeless situations into positive well-being.

Broaden the Picture to Include Others

There are so many in our communities who are lonely because their mobility is impaired. A family may have moved in across the street and do not know anyone in the neighborhood. Another's neighbors who had become best family friends had received an overseas appointment, so they now find themselves bereft and very lonely. These are people whose lives have shrunk around them. Each has feeling of isolation and abandonment. Their need becomes obvious to them as well as to an observant pastoral mind.

Even the best intentioned pastoral person cannot personally fill all the missing gaps that occur in our society and provide the advice, company and fellowship such people need. However pastoral support can be proactive on their behalf.

Pastoral visitation is a means by which a sensitive visitor can elicit something of the likes and skills, the preferences and the objections of these lonely people. The pastoral person may be likened to a matchmaker looking to find people with related needs or possess necessary gifts and bring them together.

For the elderly or those with restricted mobility, the best tonic they can receive is to be linked with other people with whom they can identify and share common interests and backgrounds. However, it is better if the link is made outside their living environment. Even with limited mobility they may be able to be assisted to a vehicle and be taken to where they can meet regularly with others in similar circumstances and, therefore be, an understanding group. It may have to be a wheelchair-friendly place. It may simply be a coffee morning or afternoon. Table games or an occasional speaker may be able to make the gathering more interesting and varied.

> *It is by constant encouragement from a pastoral person that this healing is able to continue and even be hastened.*

For those where former links of friendships have been broken, the pastoral person may have the opportunity to help them forge new links with other individuals or families of like mind or similar circumstances. The ability to identify needs, interests, create opportunities to broaden the horizons for the lonely ones, help them make new contacts and so form new alliances of friendship and support is pastoral care.. This enhances and facilitates the further ministry of the church.

Softening the Severity of the Situation
A person requiring pastoral support may be trying to deal with a situation which has traumatized them physically, emotionally or psychologically. We all react differently to shock experiences but these situations are always serious and painful intrusions into their lives. Very frequently it is quite unexpected, the surprise factor adds to the severity of the impact.

It may take many visits before the victim is able to feel comfortable dealing with the experience. Often, the occurrence has destroyed trust and confidence in other human beings. Reticence lingers because they remain suspicious that any form of closeness with another will lead to further hurt. The severity of the emotional and psychological hurt can only gradually be softened. It is difficult for people so injured to let their rational mind guide their thinking. A pastoral person will only succeed if they show evidence of genuine concern.

Often, these traumatized people are unable to rise above their mental confusion without a constant reliable source of support and knowledge. Such pastoral support must be there without conditions, at any time, so that the severity of the pain can be relieved, without such help the condition may lead to a nervous breakdown or worse. Some may need to be directed to a professional for traumatic stress counseling or more seriously for psychotherapy. The pastoral person in these cases needs to know his or her limitations. A build up for any recommendation for a referral is necessary. Any reassurance must confirm that their condition, though it may be remedied, may require this specialist help. If pastoral support is withdrawn during such therapy, the troubled one may think it has been withdrawn because of some stigma attached to this condition. The patient will need to be reassured that while receiving this specialist help the pastoral person will continue to be available. Any loss of contact at this stage would only complicate the problem increasing the patient's depression and mistrust.

> *A pastoral person will only succeed if they show evidence of genuine concern.*

The pastoral person needs to be alert to the differing needs, in such cases, if his task of assisting to relieve the severity of the situation is to be achieved.

Strengthens the Body and Mind for Action.

Any serious upset to the normal routine is likely to affect a person's physical functions. The gastro-enterinal system may react with constipation or diarrhea. Stomach disorders may be evident, accompanied by stomach cramps and frequent retching. The cardio vascular system reacts with chest pains, while tension may generate frequent headaches. The skeletal system makes itself known by joint pains or general body aching. Any or several of these disorders can lower the person's ability to concentrate on current work or perform normal duties involving physical exertion.

The alert pastoral person can, with experience, assess whether the physical problems he or she observes require a medical opinion or possibly either medical and/or psychiatric treatment.

Where these are not necessary the pastoral person will try to turn the mind of the patient off the trauma onto more positive thoughts and activities. Recognition and acceptance, of what the anxiety and stress is doing to them, often, leads to a concerted effort to deal with the problem and therefore to strengthen the body and the mind. This starts the process of healing the psychological wounds. Such healing enables a return to a normal healthy life.

It is by constant encouragement from a pastoral person that this healing is able to continue and even be hastened.

Lifts from the Slough of Despondency

The majority of us living, in the Western world of capitalism and globalization with all its ills, expect employment, health, education, social benefits and leisure time as their rights. For many their slogan might be, "maximum benefits for the minimum of effort." We have come to accept as necessary an amazing range of goods and services supplied by this technological age and State welfare provisions. When our normal routine and comfort is interrupted by adversity, we are devastated. For many it is such a new experience, that they are overwhelmed by despondency and depression. The high rate of youth suicide in western countries is because young people are not able to access the way of life they feel has been promised them or are chastised by those in authority, family or society generally for inconsiderate or anti-social behavior which arises from this sense of being denied by society. They may be unable to perform or compete in their world and have missed out on the real opportunities that they expect life to provide without significant effort on their part.

It is not only young people who are overtaken or lose their way when their reasonable expectations of life have some bitter interruption, with some significant effect upon them. The pastoral person may be called to help such people.

> *It is not only young people who are overtaken or lose their way when their reasonable expectations of life have some bitter interruption . . .*

In such cases, avoid the obvious order to "snap out of it." This may well be the logical thing to do but it will not meet the psychological need of the situation. It can only bring an antagonistic alienation. These people are hurting badly. They are sure no one understands their predicament. They have no guide or direction for their future, feel lost and helpless unable to see or think rationally.

The use of an authoritarian direction will only cause further doubt and despair. They require a gentle strong hand to reach out to them but that they must accept it. There must be movement both ways. The strong hand must reach down and the weak hand must reach up.

Pastoral persons would be wise to see themselves as an understanding shepherd able to reach down, bend their knees and stretch out their hand in assurance and hope. The despairing one will respond more often to the sincere gesture of empathy and friendly help.

The Resource for the Pastoral Person

Jesus, before he finally left his followers, said that he would leave with them another Comforter. That word 'another' is a key word. Jesus was indeed a Comforter to all who drew close to him desiring comfort. Jesus' departure meant that another Comforter would need to come into the lives of believers and be their strength and counsel

He was referring to the Holy Spirit which entered the lives of the believers on the day of Pentecost. That Holy Spirit not only provides comfort to believers, it is this spirit which gives power to those who are responsive and desire to be comforters to others in the name of Jesus. Jesus sets before us the supreme example of the shepherd – the one who committed to us this ministry to others in need. The Holy Spirit makes us aware of the way and the method Jesus would use if he were in our shoes in any particular situation.

It is the Comforter within us that turns human caring love into a divine caring love for the hurting, the needy , the bewildered, the lonely, the grieving, even the unlovable outcasts and those on the outer limits of society. The Holy Spirit is the greatest resource the pastoral person can draw upon as he or she sits alongside the person to whom they are ministering with love, care and hope for their recovery.

CHAPTER 2

Questions When In Crisis.

When bad or hurtful things befall the good, the not so good or anyone else, there are some questions which inevitably torment the mind such as : "Why Me?", "Why this?", "Why now?" "Where to from here?" Other pressing questions may arise depending upon the nature of the crisis or tragedy and the circumstances of the sufferer. These are important questions, and, unless satisfactorily dealt with, are likely to produce an anxious state causing psychological as well as physical problems. Notice the first three have negative connotations. Questions in crisis are usually negative.

These questions also indicate there is a strong element of grief in the situation. The word 'crisis' suggests a personal threat – perhaps, humiliation or a loss of an accustomed way of life or familiar conditions. Clarity of mind may have been one of their notable characteristics involved. They are now having difficulty to concentrate, think logically or organize their priorities aright. The crisis has noticeably damaged their smooth functioning and internal world. Even when they become angry over theirs or someone else's folly or carelessness, that anger may be ill-directed or hysterically out of proportion to what has occurred. Except for the question relating to the future, the other questions have complications of innocence, resentment and surprise at the outcome of events. Very often, a crisis and the mental turmoil over what has happened, prevents restful s leep which further increases their inability to think clearly and rationally.

These questions may indicate a serious need for some pastoral intervention or personal awareness of spiritual need and understanding of the way that divine resources are available in resolving the effects of the crisis.

Why Me?

This question denotes the personal involvement of the questioner with the situation. The reasonably composed and sedate life has been interrupted, disturbed, upturned and even become chaotic. It can affect one or more of the individual's or the family's life. Justly or unjustly, the character, integrity, or even career has been threatened or seriously questioned. The size, seriousness or nature of the event rousing the question is not the issue. The impact upon the life of the pleader provides the criteria for assessing the seriousness of the question.

> *The question, "Why me?" although a negative enquiry, echoes an inner belief and conviction that an injustice has been done.*

The smashing of a four year old's doll by an older brother can be as devastating to her as the death of a teenage brother or sister. An illness or incapacitation before a final examination may have as great an impact as the loss of a job by a middle aged man at a time of high unemployment. Whatever the experience, this is a question that needs to be dealt with.

The question, "Why me?" although a negative enquiry, echoes an inner belief and conviction that an injustice has been done. Of all the hundreds of cars returning from holidays on the motorway, why was my car the one to be hit? I am an innocent party. The car in front and behind could easily have been involved. Why me?

Could there be anything seemingly more unjust than the birth of a congenitally malformed child or the diagnosis of breast cancer to a young woman pregnant with her first child? This question in such cases takes on the mood of despair, anger and a sense of sabotage of their most cherished aspirations. Why Me?

Self Pity Will Not Help

To persist, reflecting and adopting a self-pitying mode, which the question implies, only exacerbates and even distorts the whole set of circumstances. To prolong the ordeal by dwelling on this question turns it into an obsessional mental preoccupation to the exclusion of more productive thoughts and activities. To hover over this question like an eagle over its eerie full of hatchlings and not search for their food only starves the mind of any motivation to continue living. In other words to immerse oneself in self pity is not helpful.

The "feel sorry for yourself" gloom is what this question indicates. The self-pity syndrome exposes a closed mind which can only see the crisis and its most dire consequences. This cry is one big lament for what was and what should be in their eyes.

After any accident the police and fire brigade clear up the accident site to restore the flow of traffic. If there has been any toxic or hazardous spills including fuel, they are washed away so as not to cause any further accident or injury. By maintaining this question at the top of the mind; the crisis is revisited in its messiest state. It is like the injection of an anesthetic to numb all feeling against other new positive influences, or allow any readjustment to normal life. The evidence at the crisis scene at its most horrendous remains uncleansed.

What is achieved by visiting those road side crosses for years, to place flowers where a loved one or friend was killed? Any true resolution of the grief of death of anyone is accomplished when they are able to resume life fully without the constant reminder and the influence of the departed over their lives. The memory of the deceased may be cherished without being slavishly tied to such a long term memorial ritual. Such practices keep resurrecting the dead in the minds of the living.

The "Why me?" question may be similarly applied. While that question is active in the mind, the influence of the crisis is never allowed to be forgotten nor permission given to set off in a new direction.

Why Not Me?

Instead of the question, "Why me?" another more potent attitudinal question is "Why not me?" That alters the whole approach to the crisis. It lifts the burden of feeling sorry for oneself from the mind.

Crises are occurring innumerable times every second to people throughout the world. The odds against anyone going through life trouble free; cruising along without problems and trauma-creating episodes are astronomical. It is logical then to review all stress creating turmoil and ask, "Why not me?" or "Have I any legitimate claim for exemption from all adversity during my life?"

An obvious response to such reasoning is to accept any crisis as one of those things that, from the very nature of our human existence in the world, must occur from time to time. The advantage of adopting this approach is that it offers a new approach. Many people find themselves bogged down in the morass of their troubles. By adopting this question, "Why not me", they are able to put themselves into four- wheel drive and inch their way forward to solid ground again.

"Why not me?" is the way to regroup resources and move forward. It is realistic. It affirms the belief that what is being experienced is not unnatural to human living. It is facing the situation and making personal effort to relieve the tension, make adjustments, adapt to the changed circumstances and to make positive moves equipped by the pain and struggle that has been experienced to deal with new crises; and to help others form a new understanding..

Why This?

To ask the question, "Why this? shows a need to find a reason. Some may ask it directly by asking, "What have I done to deserve this?"

Any person, Christian or otherwise when adversely affected by some crisis or difficulty seeks an explanation; that is, at least, inwardly satisfying for what has happened.

This raises the basic issues of self-pity and the sense of injustice. 'It is not fair to me' is the tenor of the first. The second aspect moves from self-pity to self- justification. 'I've done nothing to deserve this' remains stuck in their mind. They can see no justifiable evidence in anything they have done to warrant what has happened to them. The demand for a reason is to infer that there is no logical cause for it. They want some reason to justify the trauma faced.

It is an underlying demand to know the grounds upon which this interference with the status quo has been allowed. Not only is it a demand for an explanation, it is a declaration implying that there are no justifiable grounds created by the victim to warrant what has occurred. All of us have a degree of self-righteousness running through our thinking.

A recently convicted serial killer of young female backpackers who is also a suspect in a number of other disappearances, believes, that he has done no wrong and should not be in jail. His brothers, along with the police and a jury, are convinced that he committed the murders. This is an extreme case, yet it nevertheless is indicative of the way we think at times. We feel that we don't deserve many of the unpleasant experiences we are forced to confront.

One certain thing in life is that each of us sees the same things and events from different perspectives. One person can sit by the ocean watching the most spectacular dawn. With pen and paper in hand, an inspirational poem flows onto the paper. Just in front are several anglers with rods in hand. Their concentration is on the little tugs at the end of their lines. When they land a plate size fish, they are full of delight at the "little beauty" they have caught. The sunrise never caught their attention. The crisis may be seen by the one affected as being unjustified; acquaintances may see it as an unfortunate accident or a case of being in the wrong place at the wrong time; others may see it as well deserved.

Some people hold me in high esteem and are extremely cooperative, others are critical of some of the things I do. Some have opposed every proposal I put forward. I have had to often ask myself, "Why this?' or Why so?" In this examination, I have seen that purpose-driven enthusiasm is not always shared and often resented by some others with a different personality and gifts. Now, I try to assess their point of view more often when offering or suggesting new proposals. The enthusiasm of the presentation has to be toned down.

> *There will be some, who are not close friends, who may quote the old adage, "What you sow, you reap."*

The "Why this?", question should require us to look more clearly at ourselves to see whether in some way or another our motives may be interpreted as being egoistical grandstanding, selfish, demanding attention or a false confidence to cover for an inferiority complex. Before self-justification proceeds too far in the search for some reason, a degree of self examination needs to be undertaken.

There will be some, who are not close friends, who may quote the old adage, "What you sow, you reap." In some cases that may be true hence this question, "Why this?" may be applicable to ascertain whether this charge is pertinent to the current circumstances or not. To have a closed mind and try to prove it groundless in the prevailing crisis may be an unsustainable and invalid stance. A blinkered horse cannot see danger coming from its left or right. Close and not so close friends may be wearing blinkers as well.

The one in the middle of the situation is the only one who may or may not know their own deep down intentions and the motives behind what happened. It is only by an attitude that is not trying to justify its actions can this question be truly answered and the broader picture seen and interpreted.

Another way of taking this question seriously is to stand off and look as the situation objectively leaving aside your own involved feelings. Many have been the times I have been in the Emergency Room when a motor vehicle accident case has been brought in with severe head injuries. The patient has been rushed to theatre to have a Richmond Bolt inserted into the skull to relieve the pressure on the brain. Even so, the Neuro-surgeons were very doubtful as to the viability of future brain function. Weeks spent in a coma in the Intensive Care Unit, and then the eyes begin to flutter. Days later, the lips begin to form words followed by the recognition of loved ones around the bed. Sometime later life support systems are removed and clear speech begins to return. After perhaps a couple more months the patient is discharged with full brain function except for a little weakness down the left side.

The patient could dwell on the "Why this?"; bemoaning the loss of those four or more months, berating the driver of the other vehicle; cursing God for letting it happen; or bewailing the loss of career opportunities through the left sided weakness. In most cases of trauma or crisis the surviving sufferer should be able to survey the damage and say, "It could have been worse." The emergency doctors and surgeons gave the above patient little chance for the return of any reasonable brain function. Except for that one-sided slight paralysis the brain function has little impairment. He could have been a vegetable and I have seen many left in such a condition.

It could have been worse.

In looking at the result of the crisis, our response, could easily be, "It could have been worse." Crises may produce many different outcomes. Any survivor of a crisis has weathered the worst of the storm, which is one cause for being grateful and offering thanks. To recognize a cause for thanksgiving or any small mercy, in the midst of the chaos is to start setting life back into balance without any serious permanent psychological damage. Thanksgiving for protection from some worse fate, incapacity or hardship is one of the strongest weapons with which to fight off the effects of a critical period.

To be thankful that it wasn't worse enables a constructive approach to any readjustment, correction or other change necessary as a result of the recent disruptive period. Thankfulness is the starting point from which to enthusiastically pursue the discovery of "What's next".

Another aspect of this question is that without a period of traumatic stress, which must involve getting up off the floor, facing it and start reliving and utilizing the teaching learned from the experience, it is possible to become a soft, spineless and gutless character. Trauma is able to stiffen character, and develop the wisdom to respond to other adverse situations that will occur in our lives from time to time. Every time we are forced to take our place in the hot seat we gain immeasurably in understanding and in the acquiring of added abilities to tackle and cope with new situations which will certainly occur. Accepting that it could be worse makes us stronger to compete in life's battles.

> *Another aspect of this question is that without a period of traumatic stress, which must involve getting up off the floor,*

Many will cry out to God to overcome the crisis or immediately remove the cause. If God rescued us from every such predicament, people, we would become very weak and indecisive persons with very little stamina, fortitude and coping skills. In addition, another in difficulties might feel your intervention (offered out of little personal experience of suffering); insufficient leaving them dissatisfied-leading to a sense of abandonment by God and the church as well as isolating themselves from further efforts of assistance. We need to attempt to turn each crisis we encounter in others into a learning experience to enable us to fit more comfortably into society in aiding others to accept the reality of their situation.

If we do not let such crises become learning experiences, it can so deflate the personality that all confidence in the present or future is weakened. In other words, the depression following the crisis must be dealt with. When that is eliminated, a new strength to face and overcome remains, so that every new negative situation that seeks to suppress our buoyancy of spirit will not overcome us. This new wisdom and confidence makes possible the early detection and deflection of what may develop into a new crisis or even help us to meet it head on before any damage is done and the self and those around are hurt.

> *A crisis involves the expenditure of too much time, energy and mental activity resulting in physical, emotional and spiritual exhaustion*

"Why this?" has to be satisfactorily dismissed so that the answer to the next question "Why now?" may be addressed with enthusiasm for it may lead us to a new life, new career, new relationships, new interests with all their challenges and excitement of change..

Why Now?

We are never prepared for a crisis. We may see it as threatening, but never convenient. A crisis involves the expenditure of too much time, energy and mental activity resulting in physical, emotional and spiritual exhaustion. A crisis debilitates and drains all areas of a person's life. A crisis puts many other activities, including important ones, on hold until the predicament and its effects can be satisfactorily dealt with to allow life to continue even though it may have to change direction.

A crisis may arise in the midst of a major project, six months into a pregnancy, when recuperating from surgery, when forming a new relationship or when the spouse has walked out leaving a mountain of debts or any other unenviable upheaval. There would be few if any who would say that a crisis came at a convenient time. Because of the disruption to life and thought, along with its twin, anxiety, the question that often comes to mind is, "Why now?" None of us like an interruption to our schedules at any time. There are often things to be completed with a deadline; by a crisis, much is thrown into confusion; delays are inevitable; opportunities are lost; relationships are broken or strained; loved ones are deeply hurt or bewildered. Often this is at a time when you need their support most, and important tasks and routines, are neglected. Any or several of these together all add to the confusion. Therefore, it is a legitimate question. "Why Now?"

> *A crisis may arise in the midst of a major project, six months into a pregnancy, when recuperating from surgery, when forming a new relationship or when the spouse has walked out leaving a mountain of debts or any other unenviable*

The cause of the disarray may have arisen from outside avenues; another's carelessness, vindictiveness, an accident caused by another or a breakdown in infrastructure or any combination of these. The damage or harm may be moderate or considerable. The timing of such interruptions and intrusions will never be convenient because it interferes with life's equilibrium and smooth function. Therefore, any such circumstances will suggest the question, "Why now?"

Throughout history, death or tragedy has struck from before a birth to very old age. Nothing in life can be taken for granted. Trauma and separation never come at the right moment. Sometimes it may be sudden or unexpected, at other times; the warning signals may go unrecognized. It may be of short duration or it may be long and drawn out such as for those comatosed in a critical care unit. They may have to reorientate their lives and learn to master new skills or unaccustomed restrictions.

Death is a crisis blow that is responsible for family and personal disorientation which varies according to the nature of the relationship between family members and their past history. For a dysfunctional family, few members may be seriously affected except where the issue of family disunity raises issues of guilt and regret. Some may be relieved over the demise.

For a very close loving family the sense of loss is very keenly felt and for some, the sense of loss is never permitted to be resolved. It is carried to their grave. Such long term harboring of grief is unhealthy and has physical, behavioral and psychological repercussions.   A death in the family may raise disputes over a will or possessions of the deceased. In such cases, a family can become embroiled in a serious conflict, with some never speaking to a family member or members again. These are considered to be unresolved crises. There is never a suitable time for the crisis of death to strike except when it is a terminally ill patient or a very aged frail person. Even then, the measure of grief experienced is never welcome. The need to bear the brunt and anxiety of the death of a dear one never occurs at an opportune moment. Many people are busy or too involved with their own affairs to want to share in so painful a period.

However, we should need not be as fatalistic as the writer of Ecclesiastes (3:1) who suggests that everything happens as God chooses. We cannot blame God for the predicaments in which we find ourselves from time to time. However, in these troublesome occasions when our routine is interrupted and out bodies and minds are injured by the events of the crisis it is time to seek God's comfort, wisdom strength and patience for the occasion. It is God's nature to be on standby at a time of trials and disasters. A time of crisis is like us going through the maze and out again into the open fields, perhaps, of new opportunities and to continue life's journey.

Let me suggest a strategy for any unpleasant and unwanted interlude that confuses and adds stress to life:

- ❖ Start believing now that the crisis can be overcome.
- ❖ Believe and trust that God is able to reconcile the problem and the damage as we show our trust in Him and make appropriate decisions.
- ❖ Now is the time to start repairing the situation. It may require us to seek forgiveness from another or offer forgiveness to another. Stubborn pride is not a help.
- ❖ Believe, that with the Holy Spirit's help it is possible to love the initiator of the crisis even if it hits home personally. Crisis grief can be turned into personal blessing and enrichment through the Holy Spirit's help.

Why now? – No! Now is the time to be allied with God to be restored and rise from the ashes of the crisis and march forward.

Where to from Here?

The crisis puts on hold many future plans that present far reaching consequences for self and others. Illness, a death, serious injury or a broken relationship can change situations overnight or reduce us from being fiercely independent to helpless dependence. Many skills and capabilities may be stripped away. All sense of dignity is destroyed as assistance is needed with personal hygiene. The questions, already, examined, seem small compared with the broader picture as the future comes into focus. The question now becomes "Where to from here?" Perhaps career, marriage, family, sporting or normal recreational activities have all to be reassessed. The future may look as bleak as it can get. Those inspirational dreams of the future seem to have vanished without a trace.

It is becoming evident that close friends are not calling as often. The social circle is shrinking. To visit is too depressing. The same cheery, convivial person that friends knew is somehow hidden behind some cruel twist of life. Associates find it difficult to face the situation as it is. It becomes obvious that this could also happen to them.

The question, "Where to from here," means facing the very real possibility of a changed future. The threat being faced is that previous interests, activities and pastimes may have to be changed or abandoned to a greater or lesser degree. If we continue to speculate in negative ways about the future this can lead to depression and a general feeling of unhappiness about the future. Such feelings can easily become a permanent way of thinking and affect all of life. Efforts of recovery may be stifled or even stagnate.

It is God's nature to be on standby at a time of trials and disasters.

Where to from here? Is the question that must be encouraged to be the focus of the sufferer's mind.

Oxygen for the Climb.

These questions all revolve around something that is happening or has happened. It is an event that cannot be undone. The circumstances resulting from this eruption in life can only be repaired or remade by acknowledging that what has happened is reality and that there are years of new days, new experiences, new joys and new mountains ahead to climb. The recent crisis may or may not be life's Everest. One sure fact of life is that there will always be interruptions to the routine and course of life from time to time.

We can let the Himalayan peaks that rise along the road of life deprive us of oxygen. The wise will ensure they have their own oxygen supply to accomplish the ascent to the summit and the descent down the other side. Each successful venture further equips the pilgrim with greater balance, confidence and wisdom to continue the journey.

How can we prepare for similar emergencies in the future? Where do we find this oxygen supply?

In this modern world, we are so busy and preoccupied with career, studies, striving to maintain living standards that many things of life pass by unnoticed. My life was blessed because I came home from school to sit and talk with my mother about what happened at school and what she had done that day. We might even throw in pieces of news that we had heard or read on the radio or the newspapers. The family on a Saturday afternoon would be in the garden mowing, weeding, planting and talking together. In season we would race out of each morning to see who would be the first to enjoy the new blooms and the colors of the pansies or other spring or winter annuals as they came into bloom. Around the kitchen table, in the garden and at other times we learned to appreciate the beauty and the delicacy of God's handiwork.

One sure fact of life is that there will always be interruptions to the routine and course of life from time to time.

From as early as I can remember, it was a joy to recognize "the Windows of Wonder" (Daniel O'Leary's term from "Prism of Love"), or the little miracles that are to be seen around us every day. We need to take every opportunity to draw back the curtains from the eyes to see and reflect upon the beauty to be seen about us. As we do this the great and majestic wonders of His creation will cause us to stand in awe of God's love and provision.

To have the sharpness of spiritual eyes appreciating all of life in its fullness; to daily look out of these "windows of wonder" is to be equipped for the dizzy oxygen starved heights of any looming mountain needing to be conquered.

In the depths of chaotic and tragic despair, we should cry out, "Where to from here?" Look out of the "windows of wonder" and observe the smaller and bigger miracles to be seen all around us. Look at the works of Divine hands, and draw the confidence to grasp resources in the crisis. It is the oxygen to strengthen and encourage when we are gasping and panting for breath on the mountainside of adversity. Until the lungs are again filled with the thoughts and inspiration of His power and possibilities there is little incentive to vigorously struggle on.

Remember these miracles, are from the hand of God. Recognizing the reality of those miracles enables us to draw closer to God to infill, inspire, encourage and infuse faith to accept that He can deal with whatever attitude that weakness that may develop. He is able to fill the lungs of the mind with fresh and vital oxygen; giving strength to rise to the feet and with confidence, move to the summit and start the descent to the wide open vista beyond. To believe in the miracles we daily see enables us to believe that God can open each questing mind to heal the plaguing torments. Only by seeing those fields of miracles can we rise to our feet and press on further. God provides the vision but we must act.

More than half a century ago, I trekked in the Himalayas. My eyes saw an amazing miracle. As it was spring, the snowline was receding. Under the snow as it melted were green tufts of lush herbage. The shepherds moved their flocks of sheep and goats, higher and higher as the snow retreated. Their animals were feeding on the best. They were all healthy and plump. God never leaves us without hope. The present is left in His hand to guide so that we will be nourished with hope for each and every event that may come our way in the future. Underneath the snow of the mountain is this miracle where all the needed sustenance is provided and waiting to be used.

> *Life is for living, not moping around thinking of what might have been.*

Beneath the show of anger, confusion, heartache and disappointment lies such a miracle. It is not the time to ask, "Why me?', "Why this?", "Why now?" Rather the question is, "Where to from here?" Move forward, the sun is melting the snow to provide a better future. Those negative questions have been turned to positive answers. There is a new air of optimism. The lungs are full of this fresh air and the new strength comes with the provision for this need. The summit of this dreaded mountain becomes visible and we can visualize and enjoy the anticipation of the warmth of the sun-drenched plains on the other side.

Recognize there is a God who scatters small and sometimes bigger miracles along the way each day, to rally us in our climb. Life is for living, not moping around thinking of what might have been. Life is for marching into the future. We cannot move easily forward at a steady pace while there are our negative questions still dangling from the shoulders to impede progress.

There have been many starting out in life or were in the midstream of life whose ambition or successful venture has been cut short by accident or illness. The easiest option is to curl up in the fetal position and despondently just let the world roll by. Their misery becomes their life.

However, many when challenged by the nature of this question, "Where to from here?" are able to lift their sights to see not a sunset but a dawn throwing its light upon new directions and possibilities.

Colleen was a stay at home wife of Fred who had a very successful accountancy business. Colleen liked to pamper Fred when he came home from the office with the most exotic and varied range of delicious meals. It was always special. She would say, "A man works hard all day and needs the best when he comes home." Their marriage was very successful because they were always considering each other.

When Fred died of a sudden and unexpected heart attack, Colleen's world tumbled around her. She could see no hope for herself. Her sense of helplessness and isolation increased as many of her married friends started to lose interest because she was still somewhat attractive and now a single woman.

She began to take stock of the situation. There was no incentive to stay at home and cook nice meals for herself alone. Beside she had lost her appetite for eating. A form of the question, "Where to from here?" began to exercise her mind. She looked at her talents and what she could do. She had not worked outside the home since she was married. Just what could she do? All she could claim was that she was a good cook. "What is possible in the cooking line?" was a question which kept reoccurring. After probate had been settled she had a certain amount of money and cooking skills.

In the paper she noticed an advertisement that was looking for a chef to join as a partner in a respectable restaurant with potential. Her enquiries showed that she was the type of person they were seeking. Some of the probate money put into the partnership meant that the business could expand. Colleen would supervise the kitchen, the menu and the cooking as well as being more hands on in the preparation of the special gourmet aspects of the menu. Her many books on cooking from around the world she had collected were now kept in the restaurant's kitchen. Within a decade Colleen was a celebrity cook and the restaurant became renowned for its cuisine.

Where to from here? For Colleen it was a brilliant new life and career – a far cry from the stay at home suburban housewife.

Another person who faced that question in a similar way is the now well known motivational and inspirational speaker Joni Erickson Tada who broke her neck in a diving accident as a very young woman. Joni has traveled the word uplifting others by her willingness not to be defeated by these questions when she faced her crisis. Still severely disabled she is one of the best examples of a positive response to this question.

Joni could not have faced it alone. Along with her supportive Christian friends she sought God's help in her crisis. She has proved once again to the world that even when, in the bleakest, deepest well of despair, God was able to open up undreamed of new horizons and service to her fellow humans that would otherwise have remained untapped and concealed for eternity. Instead Joni found peace and new direction through letting her God and Savior share her load in her time of crisis.

Where to from here?

Did not Jesus say "Come unto me, all you who are tired from carrying heavy loads, and I will give you rest." Matt. 11:28 (GNB)

CHAPTER 3

A GRIEVING PARENT.

Forty years ago, in the area of the Third World where I worked for nearly two decades, almost every home would claim that they had lost through death, at least half of the children born to them, before the age of five. The main killers were malaria, either the malignant or cerebral forms; cholera, typhoid and to a lesser extent dysentery had a share in these statistics. The parents were grateful if they had three or four surviving offspring. There was an air of enduring sorrow and sadness but with an acceptance that it was a normal part of life. The figures have improved considerably by the beginning of the 21st century.

In the western world the death of a child is a uniquely devastating trauma for the parents and other siblings. The death of a person before middle age is considered outside the norm and does not conform to the accepted life cycle and expectancy. Therefore the death of a child for whatever reason is a major tragedy in the life of a family. We shall look at the needs of parents who have lost a child in early years and then for those whose child died as a teenager and older. Parental reactions vary according to the age of the child at death.

When an offspring dies, for the parents, it is a reflection of something far greater. Part of something that possibly starts many thousands of years ago has been lost. The child contained genes and DNA which goes back beyond the first forebears of the clan. This is seen with Jews and Arabs who are of Semitic origin. More than this, modern science has proved that they have an original common ancestry, as all Jews and Arabs carry a similar DNA. A child carries the DNA of both parents which have been passed down for thousands of years. So the death of a child represents the loss of a part of both parents. A parent cannot escape the fact that a part of them has died with their child.

Some hereditary characteristics have been taken to the grave. As a parent reflects on the person of the deceased child they recall seeing a child with some similar behavioral patterns, traits and nature of themselves and the other parent. This is one of the factors which makes the loss of a child so painful and real. Even if the child was rebellious, disrespectful, a social misfit and has given a bad reputation to the family name, these are all forgotten by most parents as they grieve. Although death may have occurred by road accident, suicide, overdose of drugs, careless skylarking or some form of anti-social behavior the parents cannot dismiss the fact from their minds that it was their child and that a part of them died with the child.

> *The death of a person before middle age is considered outside the norm and does not conform to the accepted life cycle and expectancy.*

The relationship of the mother to the child starts from the realization that she has missed a period and is pregnant. The mother's bonding with the child, except when the child is unwanted or unplanned, continues to grow as she feels her body changing. The father's bonding and attachment often increases noticeably with the baby's quickening and the first movements in the womb are felt. The feeling of fetal activity impresses upon him the reality a living being of his making. The parents are able to share their stronger feelings about the child fantasizing their desired future for and with the unborn child.

On the death of the child those pre-birth fantasies and aspirations which continued to be recalled and nourished are now sadly confronted by the new reality. There is a measure of disappointment, pride, regret, joy, thanksgiving or other feelings depending on how the child was developing up to the time of the demise.

Then there are the parents whose child was unintentionally conceived. The unwanted pregnancy caused friction with the grandparents for many reasons: stopping of education, the sacrifice of career opportunities or being forced into a marriage to save the family name. Each of these disastrous possibilities leaves a nasty taste of bitterness and regrets so the death of the child may bring a sense of relief for the mother and the father. Even that cannot stop the sense of loss because attachments have been formed from conception to death. In fact, that relieved feeling may also be for the child, who escapes an unfortunate life resulting from inadequate parental bonding, poverty or an uncertain future.

That sense of relief adds further ammunition to the arsenal of guilt harbored since the conception. It all was a mistake from the beginning and this only compounds it. In such cases there is a need for someone to spend time with both parents allowing those feelings to be exposed, forgiven and gently forgotten. Life should be lived without such a cloud out of the past, possibly a teenage mistake, overshadowing every move they make in the future.

Pre-mature death in infancy or earlier

A 21 year old expectant mother and her husband rang for an appointment. When we met she was in the third trimester and very anxious.

When she was fifteen years old, she fell pregnant to her boy friend who was eighteen years of age. Both sets of parents were hostile and aggrieved over the pregnancy. United, they insisted on an abortion against the wishes of the girl and the father. The abortion was duly carried out. As soon as Julie was eighteen and had left school, she and Charlie were married. Now twenty-one, she was expecting again.

The reason for their call was because over the last five years she had periods of suicidal urges. This new pregnancy had deepened her depression, bringing the matter of the abortion to her mind repeatedly. She had been to the minister of the protestant church they attended, who had a strong evangelical point of view. He called her sinful for such thoughts of suicide, needing to repent and seek God's forgiveness for clinging to those urges. This only made matters worse, heaping more and more guilt upon her. This caused her to relive the abortion episode all the more.

After her visit to the abortion clinic, what had happened there was a taboo subject never to be raised again in either of the parental homes. The grandparents' residual judgmental attitude never waned. As far as they were concerned it was disgraceful and a closed subject. To make matters worse, at the time of the abortion the fetus was twenty-one and a half weeks. The medical officer, presumably under the influence of the grandparents, recorded it as being 19 weeks. According to law any birth beyond 20 weeks gestation has to be registered, named and a proper disposal of the body arranged. This fetus recorded at 19 weeks was considered a non-person so no name was given to it. For Julie and Charlie the unborn child was a person, a being made of their union. Julie was not allowed to see the fetus and it was dumped into the trash bin for the hospital's incinerator. Julie was not allowed to grieve for the baby and had to go back to school. The minister sided with the grandparents that the fetus was not a person. Not to have a name only made the matter worse. During their first visit, it was made clear to Julie and Charlie that the aborted fetus was their child and they could grieve for their loss. We started by giving the baby a name. This was to allow them to recognize and honor this person, their own baby and start to grieve for a five year old event; this was a tonic to their minds and spirits. For Julie, the sense of relief was very evident in my office that first morning. The cloud of depression was lifting and a few weeks later she had a normal delivery of a healthy girl. Not another suicidal thought crossed her mind.

More than ten years later my pre-retirement assignment was to set up a Chaplaincy Department in a hospital in a town some seventy or more miles away. Living in the district were Julie and Charlie, very happy, with three more children. Julie was the founder and leader of a Christian dance group which performed at church services in the area. She provided all the interpretive choreography. It was a radiant happy mother, with a deep spiritual understanding and experience.

With the loss of her child being recognized she was able to grieve, mourn and finally say good bye to that fetus. This was done openly in my office and much more so in the privacy of their own home. Julie, I am sure, would have committed suicide before she delivered her child – her second.

For many, the loss of a child by miscarriage, still-birth, as a newborn or preschool child needs to be acknowledged as traumatic as the loss of a husband or a parent. Time must be given to grieve and complete the need to say goodbye in the most appropriate way for the parents. Remember your way might not be their way. In Julie's case she had to be relieved of all the guilt, shame, and stigma heaped upon her by both families and the church. She also had to be allowed to accept that she was still loved by God who understood and forgave her. Above all, she also had to be able to forgive herself, even though the decision for the abortion was not hers. Julie and Charlie had to grieve their loss, irrespective of the circumstances.

> *Time must be given to grieve and complete the need to say goodbye in the most appropriate way for the parents.*

Having been heavily involved with the pediatric oncology and pediatric cardio-thoracic surgery units it was a privilege to sit alongside of parents as they feared the worst and in many cases experienced the worst for their infant child. No matter how young the child, it is essential the parents be allowed to recognize the immensity of their loss; to express it openly and in private and to know that they have the support of others in their grief.

One Lebanese mother had new born twins. One had a serious, congenital heart abnormality and was awaiting open heart surgery at the age of 5 days. The mother treated me coolly, expressing her anger at the unfairness of God to allow this injustice. It was suggested that she should tell God exactly what she thought of him calling him all the "b…. so and sos", if that was how she felt. She was told that God would not think it blasphemy and would understand what she was going through.

Next morning, the day of the surgery, I went into the unit and was greeted with a smile and an excited saying, "I did it, I did it. I called him all the names I could think of and it made me feel good." The child went to theatre and the operation was successful. A ministry of support and prayer was only possible because she was given permission to express her true feelings and anger to a caring, sensitive God who understands all our circumstances and pain. She almost lost her child but in doing so she discovered the real God who was not the wrathful vindictive God about whom she had been taught as a child. She discovered a God who was concerned for her in her crisis.

One mother's perfectly formed son was still just born before full term. It was arranged that while she was in hospital she would nurse her son each morning and afternoon for an hour. Knowing the undertaker it was possible to arrange that on the morning of the funeral the baby and the casket would be taken to the home. The body was placed in what was to be his room and on what was to be his change table. The parents dressed the baby placed it in the small casket and screwed down the lid. They then drove in the undertaker's car with the casket between them to the funeral service.

The mother remarked how she felt that her son now had a personality. He had been in his room and had become part of the home and family. This is another aspect of how pastoral care may enable the parents of a still born child to properly recognize and feel the child they conceived belonged to them. It made the resolution of their grief much easier. Years later they can still mention his name naturally.

For still-births and neonatal deaths, pastoral care should ensure that there are enough photos of the baby; a death certificate should be given to the parents; the baby has been given a name; if possible the parents should have the opportunity to be involved in post-death preparations. All of these are on the proviso that there is no major congenital deformity or other condition that may be offensive or disturbing. Although, I have seen parents view badly malformed new-borns and say how beautiful they are. Often beauty is in the eye of the beholder. At all times discretion should be used.

The loss of a child in utero, as a new born or in early infancy may be in some respects more tempestuous and hurtful than when the child is a little older. In any of these stages the infant is dependent upon the parents for daily provision, care and protection. A parent or parents, experiencing such a loss feel the weight of the responsibility and therefore have that real sense of having let their offspring down.

Guilt

Most parents feel responsibility toward their children, particularly if they are under ten years and especially for those under five years. Mary was a three years old. Her mother, Bridget, was a very protective, caring mother. Safety was almost a fetish with her. In their backyard she had swings, a see-saw, sand-pit and other play items for her children. The backyard was fenced off on both sides of the house to keep the children in. Of course the two older children could unlock the side gates.

It was 4:30 in the afternoon and Bridget had started to get the evening meal, after having checked that Mary was playing in the sand pit with some of her dolls. The other two children were with school friends. A half an hour later she heard the squeal of brakes and a bang outside the house. It was Mary. She had been hit by a car. One of the older children had not locked the side gate properly. As the gate was open, naturally, Mary had gone out to find her sister and brother. So she darted from behind a parked car onto the road and was hit.

As Mary was receiving treatment in the Pediatric Intensive Care unit, Bridget was blaming herself for not having Mary in the kitchen while she was preparing the meal. Mary's head injuries were very serious and Bridget had been warned to expect the worst. This news only intensified the feeling of guilt that was beginning to break her down. To try and put things into perspective at that stage would have been futile. It would not have registered. She was too preoccupied with coming to grips with what was happening and her own sense of failed responsibility. All that I could do was to sit with her and be a comforting presence and provide assurance that she was not alone in this dreadful time of heartache, fear, and terrified of outcomes. She had to be able to talk out her feelings of guilt and hindsight assessment of what she should have done. To have attempted, at that stage, to modify the self accusation would have demolished any hope of gaining any help from me. Yet to allow her

> *Most parents feel responsibility toward their children, particularly if they are under ten years and especially for those under five years.*

to talk about her guilt at each visit would entrench the guilt factor in her mind. At times efforts should be made to turn the conversation in another direction. To talk about the dolls she was playing with in the sandpit may help to interrupt the guilt tripping. The self-blame has to be dealt with at some stage but not too soon nor too forcefully. Sensitivity is a crucial word in all pastoral caring as in Bridget's case.

Bridget could take in very little until after the funeral and then only as a soft, gentle, sensitive intrusion so that true pastoral concern is able to register. Sometimes it may take months and even longer for one hurting like Bridget to be able to accept that they cannot possibly monitor everything their children do. She had warned the older children countless times about making sure the side gate was locked. On most other occasions they had done the right thing. Bridget was bearing the burden of the unlocked gate and its consequences. Yet to have had Mary at her feet every second of the day would not be possible. Mary, like all children of her age, must have time to discover life, its risks and learn the rules of survival, within the bounds of safety.

Pastoral support in such cases may need to continue for several months. As in other situations, the guilt will not ease until she acknowledges that it was not all her fault and that she must learn to forgive herself, as well as the other children, for what happened. Forgiveness of Mary's siblings was an essential part of the healing. That should be one of the desired outcomes of pastoral care. Such a result takes time to achieve.

Pre-Schoolers and Primary Scholars

No matter what the age of the child whether in embryo or in their teen years most parents fantasize about this special one they have conceived. In their minds eye, from pregnancy onward they envisage the child's success in all aspects of life. Those mental reveries are often very idealistic. Such projections of perfection are encouraged as they see the cherub in the childlike innocence and naivety of those preschool years. The fresh simplistic openness and trusting nature in those years will strengthen anticipations of a wholesomeness of character and achievements when the child reaches maturity.

In their minds eye, from pregnancy onward they envisage the child's success in all aspects of life.

Oh! That dreadful day when they go to primary school! "My little angel is growing up too fast – no longer a baby. She won't be the same. He will grow away from me." These thoughts fill most mothers' minds as their five year old starts school. At the school gates on their first morning can you spot the mother of a first-dayer without a tear?

The primary school child has an enquiring sense of wanting to do things for him or herself. Personalities are beginning to take a more definite individuality. It is a period of more rapid learning, development of habits and ways, forming more influential relationships that often extend into their teens. During these years, lessons of trust and loyalty are being learned.

For the parents, there will be times of disappointments and delight; times of being loved and of being resented (in a child's way). Still they are their parent's little darlings, even if at times mischievous. They sometimes seem so innocent that butter wouldn't melt in their mouths, but they can also drive a parent to the point of frustration. Children's natures even amongst brothers and sisters can differ widely. Nevertheless, in the average household each one is loved and wanted. Should they die, then the grief reactions of the parents can be very different and wide ranging.

One Sunday morning a seven year old was in the front passenger seat of the car being driven by his father to the hardware store. His father's mind was preoccupied with the house repair job he was doing and the materials he needed. He didn't see the red light and went through it without slowing down. The passenger's side of the car took the full force of the impact from a car crossing the intersection on the green light. In hospital, his son was on a life support machine. His father was charged with negligent driving by the police. The next day, outside in the corridor of the unit, while the doctors were with his son, he was pacing up and down in a violent rage, smacking his fist into the palm of his other hand saying quite audibly, "If I get my hands on the other driver I'll kill him."

It was a furious red-faced anger which kept him repeating the threat. More significant was the magnitude of his denial of what really happened. At that stage he had to shift the blame onto someone else. This angry denial was his way of reacting to a deep conviction of guilt, I suspect that the anger was against himself but, at that point, he could not admit it.

Few primary school children break the rules of accepted social behavior in most cases except possibly a child from a dysfunctional family. In these cases, the child sees, experiences or knows little of love within the family or for others. Over indulging the children is also a dysfunctional sign. This often results in the child seeking more rewards and the parents using more seductive uses of gifts to win good behavior. This encourages a child's scheming, learning to manipulate, to plot and deceive their elders to gain further advantages. When such a child dies there is a difference in parental reaction. The parent, the target of the manipulation, is more grief stricken. The child seemed to make efforts to please this parent or that was how may it now be interpreted. The other parent may have been on the other side of the deceit issuing rebukes and punishments which the other spouse would try to override or reduce. Such a child plays the parents off against each other to the detriment of the marriage relationship. On the death of the child the rift widens and the parents often separate because of different grief responses.

The loss of a child at any time may cause the parents to drift apart. This may happen where one parent wants to express the grief, while the other cannot or will not. They turn to someone outside the family for support. The pastoral advisor should be aware of the problem with a person of the opposite gender offering support to a grieving parent. The parent's appreciation and acceptance of the support sometimes may show a desire wanting to take the relationship further. This support person becomes the dependable one. This happens, particularly where the parents are unable to share their grief. The carer then becomes the surrogate caring, tender spouse which can lead to an unhealthy and unhelpful relationship, at this point. Any advisor or supporter is likely to be seen as an understanding substitute for the spouse. This is when another person should be called to take over the pastoral support.

> *The loss of a child at any time may cause the parents to drift apart.*

Death of a Teenager.

The death of a teenage child may produce a different set of dynamics. The child has moved from being a child into adolescence and is fast beginning to think and act like an independent adult. The deceased's rebellion, desire for freedom, the craving to be independent, the resentment of authoritarian figures such as teacher, church leaders and parents are factors which affect the parents' ability to mourn in a healthy way. They have mixed emotions from whitewashing all bad behavior, feeling of failure as a parent, being punished by God, to being overprotective of the other children and becoming very busy to avoid facing some of the deeper matters surrounding the death.

The nature of the parent/child relationship is a significant factor in the reaction to the death. One parent may have an inner sense of relief over the release from a bad influence on the younger siblings. The other may be regretting some aspects of the child's behavior. It is interpreted as a failure as a parent, a firmer stand should have been taken, of not being aware of the youth's problems and now it cannot be altered.

Many a time I have sat with parents of a dying teenager to hear tales of how wonderful they were, would always help anyone, so loving, thoughtful, kind etc etc. Yet interspersed with this are revelations of how he was in trouble with the authorities and was supposed to report to the parole officer the next day and now would be unable to meet his obligations.

Beside a certain roadside, there is a cross with flowers which marks the place where a young man met his death. Four years ago, this teenager was a known troublemaker and vandal. A former teacher described how he disrupted the class and would not accept discipline. One night, he was playing chicken at eleven o'clock, running across the road in front of cars and showing off in front of a group of his mates and teenage girls. He did it once too often and was hit by a car and died instantly. To the local press, his mother

> *The death of a teenage child may produce a different set of*

repeatedly reported what a wonderful boy he was, how helpful and kind he was. Another paper reported how he would race up and down the canals in a small boat shouting foul-mouthed obscenities at all the residents on the banks. The mother maintained her fiction about him until well after the funeral. He was painted the victim and the driver, an elderly woman, as the villain. The mother had to be unrealistic in her appraisal of her son because to admit otherwise was to admit her failure as a parent. Four years on her grief is still raw and she refuses to let her son go. Fresh flowers are still placed at that roadside cross.

The loss of a teenager may well devastate the whole family. Even where sibling rivalry was strong there was always in one way or another some sense of sibling bonding. The interaction between them was all part of the honing of their lives in preparation for full adulthood. The death has stripped them of an integral segment living in the community of the family. Their lives were made richer for the familial interaction and sparring with their deceased brother or sister. Siblings of whatever age should be included in decisions about the funeral service, the wording on the headstone or plaque, the disposal of the deceased's clothing and personal effects. It is at such a time as this, at any age, that they need to feel to be part of an assured they are an important member of the family. Siblings are vulnerable to any suggestion of slight or of not being as important as others in the family. In some respects they are in need of much more care than the parents, as they may be facing the issues of life and death for the first time. The focus is often upon the parents and the children may somehow slip into the background.

A young teenager was hit by a car and killed in front of her home. She had twin brothers aged eight. They were in shock, bewildered, and confused. The sister was dead on arrival at the hospital. I spent more than an hour with the boys in their home and I urged the parents to arrange with the undertaker, for a private viewing of their sister. On the Sunday afternoon, they saw their sister in the casket at the Funeral Home. One of the twins beautifully remarked, "Mummy, Jenny always wanted to be an angel" That was the image of his sister that helped him in his time of grief. After the funeral service at the crematorium I noticed that everyone was around the parents and the boys were standing by themselves. I went over, took their hands and walked them around the memorial gardens explaining to them that Jenny's ashes would be placed by a rose tree and her name would be on a plaque at the base of the bush. Those two boys were able to resolve their loss without adverse repercussions, because time was spent with them; they were given permission to air their feelings and were led to understand death, their grief reactions and their situation with greater clarity.

When a teenager or other member of the family dies, the younger children are in need of similar support, love and inclusion as the parents. When a teenager dies, their younger siblings often see them as hero or villain. The visitor should try to find out the nature of the relationships within the family, and then with gentleness help them to understand what has happened.

The affect of a teenage death can be more shattering because it is at a time of their lives when their talent and potential are beginning to emerge and the hopes and aspirations of what they may become in life are beginning to take shape. The loss of that potential, the denial of their career prospects, and the promise of their productive fruitfulness has all gone. Dreams remain dreams. Such is the nature of the feelings of those who have lost a loved teenager.

Whatever the circumstances, whoever the survivors, the need is there for sensitive people to be available to them with pastoral support. The main purpose is not to offer religious platitudes, but to be there as a comforting presence and with words of assurance and hope to suit their situation.

In a normal, healthy family where love and day to day experiences are shared openly, the loss of a teenager is severely felt. The son or daughter may have been a good student; conscientious in all that was attempted; was goal oriented and had fixed ideas on a definite career plan. The family pulled together as a harmonious team. Now a loved part of this unit is gone. The loss is devastating to every member of the family. Each made their own contribution to the family unit. Now a cog is missing. A feeling of loss and emptiness is intruding into each life. The dynamics of the family can never be the same again. Certainly, each surviving member will be supportive of each other as they share their tears and their memories. Yet they need some outside involvement otherwise they will turn inward on themselves and remain deep in their sorrow making little effort to move to higher ground. They need encouragement to see that the lost one would prefer them to live their lives fully as before only this time without his/her input and influence. The best way for them to honor their lost one is to strive to do their best in whatever pursuit they are involved. Gentle pastoral care provides support that enables them to share their memories, helping them adjust their lives to the loss.

The combinations of grief reactions within one family at the death of a teenager are many. Some deaths of an older teenager are premature due to their desire to be involved in adult pursuits to give a false impression of maturity as a member of the adult world. These engagements include many such things as over indulgence in alcohol, drugs, sex, and the thrill of fast cars and motorcycles. In spite of parental warnings, many will seek the excitement such reckless behavior gives. This compounds the hurt when the police knock at the door with the news. Then start the 'if onlys."

The question differs from those who have lost a child through illness whose mind is full of the word, "why?"
The pastoral person needs to be aware of the variety of grief reactions likely to be encountered when a child or sibling has died.

A young teenage boy was abducted, which made national headlines and an extensive search was initiated. The case received exceptional publicity actively stimulated by the parents. They mortgaged the house and raised money to perpetuate the search.

This reaction in many ways is understandable. They have many heart-rending questions and fears. What happened? Is he dead or alive? If dead how did he die? Where is his body? They are unable to bring closure to such tormenting questions. So 10 years later, they still continue to seek tangible evidence in the hope it will give them some release. Their demand for answers and their unwillingness to accept the reality that their son is probably dead keeps their grief fermenting and not allowing them to reengage in normal living with their other three children and life itself.

For those who have lost a child and have no clue as to their whereabouts or condition, pastoral or other professional care is necessary for any hope of resolution of their grief. Realistically, but subconsciously, they accept their child is gone; consciously they refuse to accept it. Their need is to rediscover a mental and spiritual ability to accept the obvious fact. The siblings would be justified in thinking that they were not loved as much. These grieving parents traveled all over the country leaving the brothers to be cared for by others as they distributed pamphlets about the abduction around every State. Because one child has died all other members of the family should not have to unnecessarily suffer. The responsibility to love and care for the other surviving members of the family should not be lost sight of. They are also grieving and are not being permitted to receive any respite or help from their grief. In their own grief these other children need extra love care and nurture from their parents in particular to deal with that grief.

Such parents need an experienced bereavement counselor preferably with a pastoral approach. A psychiatrist is not necessarily the most suitable unless spiritually perceptive. The parents in this case probably have underlying theological problems which prevent their anger and bitterness from subsiding. Their siblings attend a church school and the parents appear to have active connections with the parish. The parents turned to the church for prayers. A special memorial service in the church was held. So no doubt their questions may include, "where is God? why did God allow this to happen? or why doesn't God answer?" The remaining family members need a pastoral counselor to deal with the unresolved theological issues hindering their grieving processes.

Death of an Adult Son or Daughter.
The death of an adult child may hit a post middle-aged parent as a traumatic event or experience i.e. sudden death or an anticipated death

because of an illness. The former are generally due to accidents or unexpected cardiac arrests or strokes.

Sudden or accidental deaths give the parents no warning so the shock factor is greater. There is also the initial reaction or denial or disbelief. Where the accident is due to someone else's carelessness or negligence then the anger/emotion is likely to quickly surface. Until after the funeral is over these two emotions are mingled with guilt over lost opportunities to complete unfinished business and say goodbye properly.

Research has found that parental reaction to the sudden death of an adult child results in greater depression and guilt with accompanying health problems than those of parents whose adult child's death is anticipated over a long period of illness. The inability to bid meaningful farewells in person hurts them deeply. Farewells, at the funeral service are insufficient. In many cases of anticipated grief, the parents are also able to support the spouse and their grandchildren. They feel that they are of assistance and not useless. The down side of an anticipated death is that the parents often have a feeling of resentment at the pain their child had to suffer. For others it

The inability to bid meaningful farewells in person hurts them deeply.

can act as a preview of their own death promoting unexpressed and repressed apprehensions about their own future. For some parents, the death of a long term terminally ill patient is a relief. Unlike the sudden death, the child and family members are able to attend to family and other matters and say their good byes.

An adult child may die as a result of warfare. This is able to generate in the parents, a long term hatred over the futility of war. This may be initially smothered by comforters extolling the patriotism of the child. They are told to be proud of their son or daughter's sacrifice for their country. Such comfort may cause the parents to feel guilt if they show too much grief. It is possible that in this 21st century, the philosophy of unilateral interventions in another nation's affairs may cause an escalation in the bitterness at the loss of life through unjustified wars. Often the impact of death through war lasts longer and the grief is harder to resolve because it is not due to the fault of the deceased or any illness.

It should be noted in most cases that the difference in the parent/child relationship means that the mothers undergo greater stress than the fathers. The coping mechanisms of men and women also differ. The mother often feels closer because she carried the child in-utero and suckled him or her. The father adopts the stance of being strong in order to support the mother.

The dynamics of grief for older parents are often more complicated. Parents expect the norm that parents die before their children and that children bury their parents and not the other way around. Therefore, from the pastoral perspective, they need support to help them over the anger and injustice of the fact that an adult child has predeceased them as well as awakening them to their own vulnerability of a not so distant possible death. Again, in these circumstances the thought of the unfairness of this loss raises questions of why or why not me. A statement, like "I would have gladly changed places," is often heard.

The Place Of God.

It must be borne in mind that the untimely death of a child of any age before the parents frequently arouses doubt if not angry questioning of the place of God in all this. The Christian concept of God is that of a God of love, a God of good, not a god of evil. Particularly since the Middle Ages and up to the last half of the 20th century in order to win converts many sections of the church presented a God of punishment and wrath. It was a successful plan, particularly by Evangelicals, to frighten people into the Kingdom of God.

For the nomadic Semitic tribes of the Middle East like other primal people some 3,000-4,000 years ago, it was considered that a god, gods or spirits were responsible and plotted all that befell mankind. The Old Testament presents the concept of one God that rewarded good and punished all disobedience to His laws.

The stories of Jesus in the Gospels shows us the nature of a God who is caring and loving of all, even the alien woman of Samaria, the merciless money hungry Zacchaeus, the demon possessed, the leper, the adulterous woman and other outcasts. In fact, Jesus never condemned or turned away a needy person. He was outspoken against the self-righteous. Jesus never inflicted harm or evil on anyone. He only sought to make people physically, mentally and spiritually whole.

Where there is grief over the loss of a child of whatever age, the eternal God cannot be blamed for whatever happened. Whether it is accident or disease that has brought about this grief, it cannot be God's doing. God is ever willing to hear the plaintive cry in whatever circumstances to Him. He has given man a free will and therefore responds when we use that freewill to call upon him to support us in whatever our circumstances in life. Here it is not suggested that God will change the situation but He will support, comfort and provide for our need.

The question is frequently asked by those whose child has died, "Where was and is God in all this sadness and loss" God is to be seen in the acceptance of care offered by a pastoral person who:
- Identifies and shares the crisis with the family
- Is a present identity of trust and care
- Offers practical initiatives and provision in the home by the church. e.g. food, domestic help, guidance, contacts etc.
- Provides a clear thinking and unpressured support.
- Radiates a calming aura encouraging confidence and hope.
- Assures the interest of a caring church community to the family.

The always present God maybe found where the sincere pastoral person is able to unobtrusively and helpfully sit where they are sitting, becoming His representative presence to them. The pastoral person is the active link for the grieving back into the community of the church if God's spirit is evident in the presence of the carer.

God may also be seen and heard in the funeral service if their grief allows them to acknowledge it. This loving care does not stop with the funeral but is continues until the healing is well advanced. It is often well after the funeral service that the real quest for meaning of what happened can begin in earnest. If the carer has moved on prematurely without ensuring some follow up then to whom can the sorrowing ones turn?

Where is God when a child dies?

A human consists of body, mind and spirit. The body consists of flesh and bones and is in a constant condition of degeneration and ultimately is reduced to its basic dust-like elements. The mind, part of the body, is housed in the brain cells which also are continually dying or become damaged. The spirit is that part of the human which is the God-likeness implanted in us by God. This is a universal concept across the religions. As such, the spirit, like God cannot die. It is eternal. When a person who is a child of someone dies, his or her spirit is cherished by the God from whom it came. A grieving parent finds the true resolution of their grief when they accept that their child's spirit is in the watchful care of their God. This is the great consolation for any grieving parent.

CHAPTER 4

A TIME

TO

GRIEVE.

In modern Western society there has been a notable increase in the demand for pastoral and psychological services - the latter often requiring long-term psychotherapy. Social change, secularization and pluralism, where rituals, traditions and customs are being more and more relegated to the irrelevant, have downgraded the value of some of those practices which enabled adequate time to deal with life's crises and losses.

This especially applies where the loss involves a human life. In any disaster or major accident, trauma counselors are called into to counsel the survivors. A school child is killed in an accident; the child's class or even the whole school becomes involved in counseling. During my schooling, seventy years ago, one of my class mates was drowned. There was no need for counseling nor did it adversely affect any in the class. Our rituals, as well as, our home and societal understanding made it unnecessary.

In modern times, many grief rituals have faded from practice. Seventy years ago, a close male relative wore a black armband for three months following the death and a widow wore a black dress for twelve months to let people know they were in a mourning period and needed sensitivity in regard to space and topics of conversation. At the end of the period of mourning it was considered appropriate to continue life's normal program.

For the Jews during Aninut, (the period between death and burial), all other involvements are cancelled. During Shiva (seven days following the burial) the mourners begin to talk about their loss. Shiloshima is a period of 30 days following the burial including Shiva during which they gradually resume life in society. For one year following the death entertainment and amusements are restricted. After this, grief reactions except for brief remembrances on the anniversary are not to be shown. Jewish culture allowed for a staged movement from deep grief to the resumption of activities.[1] This time to grieve was necessary for a healthy return to normal living.

Working in the hospital, I discovered that the patient was being treated for presenting symptoms   when there was an underlying cause for the problems not being addressed. She was considered to have anorexia nervosa and was being treated for such. During our conversations we talked about her family. She mentioned that her sister was to be married in three weeks time and she hoped to attend the wedding. A casual enquiry about her future brother-in-law brought a flood of deep seated sobbing. She revealed that she was engaged to the man and six months earlier he broke off the engagement and courted her sister. Her loss of weight was not due to anorexia but the grief over a broken engagement which she could not resolve because the former beau was coming to the house several times a week. To see him with her sister kept the grief wounds open. She had no opportunity to grieve the broken relationship. She could not show it at home for fear of repercussions and accusations of jealousy. It had only one way to express itself and that was psychosomatically i.e. the mental stress of the situation affected the normal function of the body: Fortunately she was not suicidal otherwise or that would have been her other option. Grief affects people

---

[1] Lamm, Maurice, "The Jewish way of Death and Mourning" (New York: Jonathan David) pp97-141

differently. For this reason, unresolved grief is often not considered when a patient visits a practitioner with definite physical symptoms which may mask the real cause of the illness. The duration of grief can be indefinite unless it is resolved in a satisfactory manner. The manifestation of its effects can be manifold. At 10 p.m. one Saturday evening, a woman of 49 years of age was brought into the Emergency Room with a drug overdose – a suicide attempt. She was found soon after she had taken it so the stomach pump was effective. About 3 a.m. her speech was becoming more lucid. Joan had made several suicidal attempts previously and been in psychiatric units a number of times. She was currently seeing a psychiatrist.

Joan had four broken marriages. The third lasted around 18 months; the separation from the fourth marriage came after six months. The last two husbands were alcoholics. The daughter from the second marriage (her only child), who had arrived helped to fill in some of the story. Each of her four husbands was many years older than she. It did not take long before I heard that her father, whom she adored, died when she was 12 years of age, when she was going through puberty. The assumption I was able to make was Joan was searching for a replacement father figure. As frequently happens, she was considered too young to understand and be affected by her father's death. So she was pushed into the background. She was not expected to grieve and was not given time for it. She resumed school immediately and was never allowed to talk about her father. So she sought a father figure. When each marriage failed to fulfill her expectations thoughts of suicide arose and the attempts were made.

I knew her psychiatrist so I was able to ask him whether he had considered the possibility of unresolved grief. It had not arisen in his sessions with her. After listening to my observations he considered it highly likely it was so and would seek to uncover this hidden grief. There was no readmission to hospital over the next four or five years for a suicide attempt. It seems that she has been able to resolve, through her psychiatrist, in part, if not fully, her loss and the pain of her father's early death thirty years earlier.

Over the history of mankind people and cultures have developed "Rites of Passage" to deal with loss and grief. Those rites have been religious or community related ceremonies.

Mourning Rites.

We have briefly referred to Jewish mourning rites over 12 months. These rites carry specific rules for conduct when in the presence of a grieving person or their family. Like all rituals, these rites grew out of the life of the community or culture to meet the needs of the occasion. Rites not only focus upon the present, they are also intended to assist in the return of normal life. Thus these rites not only provide for grieving but aid in the resumption of life's routines. Rites over the millennia have usually been part of the culture's religious practices. They emphasize the continuity of the community and its roots as a people. The twentieth century saw change. The scientific and technological developments introduced revolutionary changes to the way society and the individual functions. In previous eras religion, with its rituals, in many respects influenced, if not dictated the way society lived and reacted to life's experiences.

In this post modern period, rituals are less practiced because many of them have failed to match the changes in society. This is no more so, than in the area of courtship and marriage. There was a courting period, the formal request for the father's permission to marry, a period of engagement of approximately 12 months then the marriage ceremony and the honeymoon. This was the accustomed ritual procedure half a century and more ago.

In this era, couples more frequently live together for some time before an engagement and marriage, if any. Now, often, the honeymoon is overlooked when a ritual ceremony does take place. The ritual of marriage in these cases has lost its true significance and in many cases is performed because as they get older they feel they should fulfill traditional expectations. Civil celebrants who often conduct these marriage rituals omit any reference to God and prayer is never offered for the couple's future. In fact, one, of the points of insistence imposed upon the celebrant is that the name of God be not mentioned.

Similarly death rites in so many cases are also being adulterated and minimized. The usual practice, half a century ago was a church or funeral home service and then a graveside or crematorium committal service, often followed by a gathering for light refreshments to reminiscence over the life and foibles of the departed. Of course, the Irish had their famous wake. It is increasingly common today to have a memorial service often in a church or home with or without the casket present. The public committal service is frequently omitted.

The Significance of Funeral Rites

The rites of death evolved to suit the needs of the mourners and the community. A death in past centuries often affected the whole of the community or class. Each member, of the clan or tribe, had their own place, function and expected contribution for the good of all. We have seen how grief can be a trap without escape unless means are provided by others to guide them out of its grasp. Rituals are able to assist in directing the grief-stricken toward a healthy resolution

- Rituals help to emphasize the change that has taken place. The community has lost a member who was integral to its life. A member of the group is now gone and therefore things cannot be exactly as they were.
- Rituals give opportunity to express deep emotions without embarrassment. The perceived role of the male is to be strong, at a death the "men do not cry rule" is able to be relaxed especially at the time of rituals. Men, women and children are permitted to express their sorrow, sadness and lamentations during and after the ritual's performance.
- Rituals are able to confirm the change in mutual relationships between the mourners involving emotions, self-image, perceptions, opinions, and the expected new contributions to the family or group. The role and tasks of the deceased have to be carried on; rituals emphasize this need by strongly stressing the loss.
- Rituals highlight the nature of the loss. However, they help to refine, also, the process of transforming the loss into

resolutions for positive reconstruction.   Rituals in stressing the reality of the loss are pointing to the need for a continuing optimistic involvement in the future.

The Functions of Grief Rituals.

Van Gennep, in his epoch making work in 1902 in categorizing of rituals saw their function as threefold: separation, transitions and incorporation.[2]

Separation.

A loved one has died. The funeral service is initially a rite of separation; it is a rite which emphasizes that the dead are no longer with them. They have to continue living without the presence and influence of the deceased. It is a rite which makes clear that there is no possible hope of their meeting or seeing each other again in this life. Before or during the rite, they may file past the open casket where the lifeless body highlights the obvious yet for many the hard to realize fact that it is the last time they will see the deceased on this earth.   The lifeless body is a stark declaration that their family member or friend is no more. The rite provides the mourners with the last opportunity to not only express their sadness but to inwardly accept that it is the last time that they ever will be in the same room or building with that human form. During the ritual or service, the concept of separation and finality is unmistakably and confrontingly obvious. There is no escaping it.

> *The funeral service is initially a rite of separation; it is a rite which emphasizes that the dead are no longer with them.*

If the celebrant of the rite tries to make it easier for the mourners by not demonstrating separation as essential to the ritual then much of the potency of the rite has been lost.

---

[2] Van Gennep, Arnold. "Rites of Passage" (London:Routledge,and Kegan Paul) 1977 p11, p 146.

My grandmother died just after my 12th birthday. I viewed the body at the service. It wasn't until they started to fill in the grave that the realization of my loss hit home and I began to cry. She was gone – separated from me.

In conducting a committal service, I tried to make the finality as realistically as possible. At the crematorium, I would leave the curtain open during the whole service and would stand facing the casket so that the mourners would also watch as the casket slid from sight. Death is final. Similarly at the grave side, I would have several spades full of soil shoveled in after the casket was lowered and before the benedictory prayer.. A funeral rite is a rite of separation, unless the mourners are led to accept this with some affect, the rite has not fulfilled its purpose.

Transition

Hertz[3] classified the death practices into three categories according to specific involvement, these are: the deceased's body, the deceased's soul and the survivors. Death rites have placed the deceased's future abode important in death rituals. Rites were performed to ensure a smooth transition into the next life. Hertz[4] tells of some Malay Archipelago tribes who have a temporary burial before the final incorporation into the future life. The Dyaks of Borneo also have a second funeral for the same reason.

The Garo People of North East India amongst whom I lived for many years have transitional rites before the soul is ushered into the final place of living which is a life similar to the present. Where a person is known to be dying, a wooden post was carved, to represent the dying person. This was sunk into the earthen floor of the verandah of the house. As the patient was dying a piece of string was tied to the big toe at one end and to this carved post or 'kima' at the other end. This was to enable the departing spirit to leave the body and find its temporary home in the kima. The relatives placed fresh food and rice beer at the base of the kima to nourish the soul so that it felt at home and cared for. This was a

---

[3] Hertz, Robert, *"Death and the Right Hand"* (Aberdeen:Cohen and West) 1960 p27.
[4] Hertz p 30ff and P 58-66.

more elaborate transitional rite, which was followed by another ritual when the spirit left the kima to enter and be incorporated in its final home.

In western funeral rites, there is emphasis upon the future life where there is a religious belief. Most have to a greater or lesser degree some concept of a heaven: most mourners see their loved one as on their way to this heaven. This belief is seen frequently in the letters R.I.P. - "Rest in Peace". Most mourners' prayers are that the deceased will have a swift and positive entry into heaven. Among Christians there is some confusion. The idea of a literal bodily resurrection at the end of the age is confused by Paul's reflection that to leave this life or die is to be with Christ which is the better option.[5] In some respects Christian funeral rites embrace what may be called a send off on the way to the future life.

Muslims are concerned that their loved ones will be able to supply the right answers to the interrogations of the angels Munkar and Nakir in the grave or 'Barzakh' (the intermediate state) before the resurrection and judgment.[6] The modernists see death as "a transitional stage in a continuous flowing process.... Death is, in fact, a rest from this troubled life."[7] Islamic writers see that the message of the Koran affirms the continuation of life. So that death is a transitional state before the ultimate rewards are issued by Allah or are incorporated into heaven or hell. Islamic death rituals are a significant reminder both for those left and those who are dead.

So whether from primitive spirit worship practices to modern world religious cultures, death and death rituals are meant to reawaken the relevance of the future life and that death is merely a transitional stage. Death rituals send the dead into this next phase of living.

---

[5] Philippians 1:23.
[6] Smith and Haddad *"The Islamic understanding of Death and Resurrection"* (State Uni. Of N.Y. Press: Albany) 1981 p 35ff.
[7] Smith and Haddad. Pp 105-106.

Incorporation

One of the most pleasing aspects of death rituals, which gives most comfort, is incorporation whether it is in the liturgy, the songs sung, the prayers prayed, the scripture read or the application of the eulogy all should involve some aspect of incorporation. Incorporation relates to the survivors as well as the deceased. For the deceased in the transitional stage of the rituals it is like the waving of farewell to relatives on a ship migrating to a new home land. Incorporation is the installation and the blessing of them in their new country; a land we might call their Shangri-La or Utopia. The concept of tearlessness, freedom from pain and stress, a territory that knows of no distress, is the place that the mourners are comfortably able to deliver them through the rituals. Those who mourn are able to take some satisfaction in having helped to deliver them with blessing into the new life. While they personally may not have achieved it, the satisfaction is in the fact that they have done what they could to fulfill their duty to their loved one and have paid their respects and endeavored to show their love.

It may be said that the typical Christian funeral rite deals with the sins of the deceased, forgiveness of those sins, separation of the soul from the body, purification of the soul and acceptance into the future life. The liturgy and prayers of many liturgical services embrace these aspects as necessary to realize incorporation into the life death.

As the dead have been incorporated into a new existence, so, the grieving loved ones   find themselves involved in changed circumstances. Situations and relationships have altered.   They themselves have to be reincorporated back into this different environment and adjust their lives to cope without the life, companionship and assistance of the deceased. The rituals should assist in this readjustment.

Normal funeral rites often are formal and adhere to liturgical formulas. They can be very cold and impersonal. The celebrant may make it personal in one segment which is called, "The Eulogy." During this personalization there is a tendency to highlight the good points of the person's character and use only bright colors in the description being painted. The reality is that in the family and with others the deceased may have been an obnoxious, domineering, officious person even if capable and efficient. A formal funeral service is expected to highlight virtues instead of realities. It often neglects to mention the role of the chief mourners in the life of the deceased. The unreal nature of the funeral presentation in many cases does not assist those left behind to express their true feelings openly for fear of being branded as irreverent and ungrateful toward the dead.

A caring pastor is able to take safeguards or cover against any false representation of the departed in the service. My endeavors to present 'warts and all' profile of the deceased often made the rite acceptable and helpful, enabling the relatives to be honest in their dealing with their grief and with each other. Such honesty frequently brought titters of laughter. In some cases, it allowed family skeletons to be exhumed, dealt with and reinterred.

The sagacity of the pastoral carer will be able to assess whether these matters need to be aired with them, after the funeral. Experience has proved that the relatives will often, raise the issues themselves and get it off their chests and allow healing of old wounds to take place and their grief to be resolved. It is known that some of the difficulties that they have been brooding over for several decades, to mention them in the presence of the deceased or other family members would have only created an uproar in the family. Such a service provides a platform for honesty. There have been cases when following the funeral for the first time it was learned that the deceased had been involved in the sexual abuse of his daughters. This has been the result of some of the other not so angelic traits of this well respected church figure being discretely mentioned in the eulogy. Without such references the victims may never have the courage to raise their own experiences. Their real grief and psychological damage may never have been confronted and dealt with.

An honest personal presentation of the deceased's life is essential if a lasting resolution of the mourners' grief is to be accomplished. Such is the responsibility of the officiating pastor. If there has been sufficient contact with the family before the funeral some indication of the family dynamics should have been noted. A good principle to adopt is never to take a funeral service unless there has been prior opportunity to meet the family. Without this much of the real meaning of the rite is not possible. How can the aspects of transition and incorporation be implemented if the deceased and the family are almost unknown by the celebrant?

Recently, at the funeral of a very very sincere Christian lady, her significant contribution to the community and the church were made known as well as the fact that she could be stubborn and impatient at times. This brought a titter and good hearted nods of affirmation. Having said that, it was possible to address the children and grandchildren and say things to them that their mother and grandmother would say as her parting words. The fact that her stubbornness and impatience was mentioned made the words to the family more acceptable and appreciated. Such was the comment of several family members after the service. In this service the family also felt that they were participants and had a real place in the rite. Also it was made more relevant because of the honest presentation of the deceased's character. The words spoken were made to feel applicable and realistic because the celebrant knew the deceased and something of the family interactions.

A funeral service becomes a meaningful rite of passage when members of the immediate family are mentioned by name. This is a good practice to adopt when conducting a funeral service. Absent relatives should also be mentioned because the fact that they were mentioned often will be relayed to them so that they will not feel as if they have been left out of this important family occasion. Their named inclusion should start with the introductory words of welcome and condolences at the opening of the service.

It is perhaps one of the sad aspects of the modern day Funeral Home where they use professional celebrants who churn out the same pat service time after time perhaps calling upon a relative or friend or two to say a few words. The only compensatory factor is that some funeral homes are engaging bereavement counselors to assist families. They are alert to the psychological dimensions of grief yet may have little or no perception of where the person is coming from spiritually. How can a spiritually unconnected therapist adequately deal with a guilt issue or the difficult situation where the deceased was a God denying wanton irresponsible person? Into what was the deceased incorporated? The therapists in dealing with such matters may denigrate any spiritual connection, raising confusing issues of faith.

A person offering a pastoral ministry as a funeral follow up, may have many spiritual issues with which they have to deal when meeting with the relatives. Without such spiritual resources being available grief resolution may be much longer, slower and more painful.

What Do Death Rites Do?
- Rituals confront the loss
- Rituals provide emotional relief in socially acceptable settings.
- Rituals enable participation in community grief
- Rituals draw together the various mourners, providing, if necessary, opportunities for reconciliations and restored contacts.
- Rituals provide a language to express the deepest feelings, sentiments and hopes for the occasion.

Sullender states "The absence of ritual and/or the misuse of ritual can contribute to unresolved grief." He sees "a direct correlation between the increased absence of ritual and the steady rise in the need for psychological services in modern society."[8]

Often the funeral service which is held a day or three after the death is not able to accomplish all of the above. At the funeral service many of the closest relatives are so overwhelmed with their loss that they cannot concentrate or take in much of what is said and done. Some just sit and stare at the casket like zombies recalling many memories without hearing many of the words uttered, except words of praise of the departed. The astute pastoral person will know that the really serious dealing with the

---

[8] Sullender R.Scott. "Grief and Growth – Pastoral Resources of Emotional and Spiritual Growth" (New York: Paulist Press) 1985 pp148-150

loss will need to come some time after the funeral. In many cases, for a healthy and comfortable conclusion to the emotional strains of the loss there may need to be a post funeral rite or two to deal with issues and make a final farewell statement.

Post Funeral Rites

Frequently, in grieving, there are deep seated emotions that are unable to be expressed openly as some others. The pastoral role is to encourage the opening up of those issues.

Some pastoral workers resort to the scriptures to try to drag out a reaction of emotional outpouring. That line may further repress those emotions even spiking further hostile feelings that then erupt over the pastoral person. An oft quoted funeral scripture, that has done damage to many a person feeling the loss of a loved one is, "Grieve not, like those who have no hope." (1 Thess. 4:13) The implication is often taken that if they show tears or breakdown, then they are telling the congregation that they have insufficient faith in the Christian hope. It can load guilt onto the loved ones so there is real danger that their grief will remain unexpressed. At many funerals of devout Christians I have heard non-family members say things like, "She was marvelous. She didn't shed a tear through the memorial service nor at the graveside. What faith!" Such comments show an ignorance and lack of understanding of the need to express the pangs of grief. Stoicism is not a trait to be proud of or espoused when a major loss has been experienced. A person who shows little emotion may be in a state of delayed shock or denial and require sensitive follow up.

The naturalness of grief should be encouraged by using the example of Jesus when he arrived at Bethany to be told that Lazarus had died. The apostle John says, "Jesus wept."(John 11:15) Who would accuse Jesus of a lack of faith in an eternal hope?

Another scripture that evokes emotion is Psalm 23. It is one of the earliest and best known scriptures, often learnt by rote in childhood by most with a Christian background. There would be few funeral services where it is not used. It is a favorite bedside scripture used by clergy with the dying. It is often associated by the hearer with earlier events in life. Such recall may relate to events in the deceased's life that had long ago passed into the memory. Scripture in evoking memories, whether good or bad, from the past is able to assist in the release of grief expressions.

A pastoral incentive to effect healthy grieving is the use of post funeral rites to encourage grief expression and release from the restrictive bonds that the memory of the departed loved one is still holding over them. These rites may be as varied as the fertile mind of the pastoral helper is able to make relevant to the case in hand.

Over a decade ago, a chapter of the Sudden Instant Death Syndrome Association invited me to conduct the annual "Remembrance Service" for members of those families who had lost an infant through cot-death in the previous twelve months. It was to be held in a park. The location decided the nature of the service I would conduct. The park was at the end of a point that stretched out into the bay. I requested that each parent bring a daisy like flower to represent their lost child.

After prayer, I related the story of a mother, I knew, who was in the Delivery Suite and in labor. Complications arose so she was rushed into the theatre for a Caesarian birth. Whilst on the operating table the mother clinically died. Her heart and breathing stopped. She said that her spirit left her body and rose toward the ceiling from where she watched what was happening. She saw them remove her dead daughter from her open womb. The next thing, she was running down the tunnel holding the hand of a beautiful young woman whom she knew was her dead daughter. The story continues but we will leave it there. Suffice to say the mother revived but not the babe.

I described, to these grieving parents in the park, how that story fitted in with Paul's words in 1 Corinthians Chapter 15: 35-58 where he describes the future post death body. How our dead bodies would be replaced with a spiritual body that would not degenerate – from a mortal body to an immortal body. I have for many years believed that our post death body would not be as a babe if we died as an infant or as a ninety-two year old if we lived to that age. Age would not be a factor in the spiritual body. Its appearance will be as in the prime of life. My experiences with other people who have clinically died have confirmed this and it is aligned with Paul's teaching. Those parents were assured that in the future life their cot death child would be recognized as a young man or woman. Thus the Christian hope was presented.

The second part of this rite was down at the waters edge where they were given four options to suit the stage of their grief. The flower they brought represented their child.

- They could find a piece of bark or something that would float, place their flower upon it and watch the flower sail away from them on the tide until it capsized or disappeared from sight.
- The flower could be cast upon the water to float off or sink to the bottom.
- Those who wanted to spend time to meditate and think upon their child, what happened and their lost aspirations, were invited to take their flower and petal by petal pull it apart and let the petals float away on the water. They could make it as long or as short as they felt they could bear.
- To those who felt they were not at the stage of releasing their child and to say their goodbyes it was suggested that they could cup the flower in their hands look upon it and its meaning. They were invited to take it home and when they felt they could, to come back and carry out one of the other three options.

For those who adopted one of the first three options, the idea was that as the flower or the petals drifted away, it was like their baby talking leave of them. It was their opportunity to say their good byes as the flower and its parts disappeared from sight.

It was interesting to observe how they each found their own place at the water's edge and each seriously carried out their choice of options. Some lingered for a half hour or more and when they felt they had completed their business with their child they silently moved off and we gathered again further back in the park for a BBQ breakfast.

The association secretary reported back some weeks later to say that many of the families were able to complete their grieving and move on from under the heavy cloud of their loss, hanging over them by really being able to say goodbye. Others expressed that they found the ritualistic exercise was able to help them face some issues that had been blocking their healthy grieving.

By contrast, there was another person who initiated her own rite to declare that her time of grieving was over and it was time to resume her normal life. This turned sour by the insensitive and uncaring remarks of her friends.

I met Peter and Betty during Peter's admission to hospital where he died. It was possible to get to know much about them during that period. They were both in their early seventies. They belonged to a seniors group which met weekly in the local Community Hall for games fellowship and singing. Both were musically gifted; Betty played the piano while Peter, with a rich baritone voice, conducted the singing.

They had been married for over fifty years and had a very loving sharing marriage. Following Peter's death, Betty grieved deeply and expressed it volubly and copiously with tears. She could not bear to go to the group meeting for several months after Peter's death. After just over six months she started going back and then one week as her rite of passage into her new life without Peter she sat down at the piano and started to play as she had done previously. Many audible "Ohs" echoed across the room. At the end of the program and over a cup of coffee several remarked to her that they did not know how she could have played the piano so soon after Peter's death. This initiated deep hurt, confusion and distress that caused Betty to make a trip to the hospital and to my office.

People need time to grieve but they also need a time to declare and show that they are resuming their life and that there has been sufficient time and emotional expression for them to have dealt with their loss. The length of time for grief varies from person to person and the nature of the relationship prior to death also has its influence. A happy relationship may require a shorter time because they have talked it over before hand or else the survivor is so devastated that they may take years to get over it or so deeply pine to hasten their own death. A bad relationship is able to have evoked so much anger and bitterness that the relief to be free makes the need for time to grieve unnecessary. The grief in such a case may also, be the grief over the lost years in a bad relationship; the bitterness may be so great that forgiveness is not possible and that wounded heart grieves for years.

Betty's many happy years left her with few regrets or negative feelings about Peter. She was thankful to God for the more than fifty years they had been allowed to enjoy together. Peter had told her not to mope around after he was gone and not to let her musical talent rust away unused. Betty had a vast store of happy memories to keep her happy and contented for the rest of her days. As we talked about all these things she could see how her getting up to play the piano was her rite of passage telling the others she was living normally once more. That rite was announcing she had moved beyond the stage of deep grief. In her understanding of it in this way her face began to light up in relief and the confusion and hurt had begun to disappear. It was also recalling happy times of sharing with Peter. Such times were filled with gratitude for those 50 years.

In our modern western world, people are not accustomed to rituals except for those people who have a background with liturgical churches. To mention the word ritual, for many, would conjure up flowing robes, candles and incense waving. Rituals can be as simple or as complex as you as you want them. For Betty, her ritual was to return to the piano where she and Peter led the group. It was a special occasion. It was not easy to do; it broke the grieving cycle.

A simple prayer, a specially focused scripture reading and reflection, a hymn or song are able to stir feelings, reveal new meanings for action, open avenues for peaceful resolution or initiate the removal of memorabilia that maintain the grief momentum. It is essential for a time to be allowed to grieve following an important loss of any sort without the loss hampering a fruitful happy life. A simple formal ritual may be needed to mark the transition to a new phase of life.

A pastoral person is in a unique position to foster, suggest or initiate a suitable ritual to suit the person and background. It must not be imposed or the grieving one may feel they must do this thing or else! With the wrong attitude a ritual is meaningless. The ritual may be a return to the place or scene closely associated with the loss and with prayer or other appropriate action closure may be possible. The rite is a symbolic act and may or may not use words in its enactment. Betty's rite did not carry words but conveyed meaning for her even if it was misunderstood by others.

Onno van der Hart[9] tells the story of Marella (21/2 years) who had difficulty in eating and keeping her food down for the previous six months. Her mother had delivered an incurably ill child and her parents spent much time at the hospital until their infant son died. The parents did not tell Marella about the death. Then suddenly

Maralla observed they stopped going to the hospital. It was from this time that Marella's eating problems began.

A Therapist suggested the parents tell Marella that her brother had died and was buried in the cemetery. Marella was also told that it was important now to bury his clothes. Her father dug a hole in the back yard of their home. Her mother neatly placed some clothes in the hole and Marella laid a pair of little shoes on top of the clothes. Her father filled in the hole and planted a tree on it. Van der Hart reports that Marella's symptoms disappeared from that day and she began to talk about her little brother. It was a family rite without a set formula, yet, it was effective.

---

[9] Van der Hart, Onno. "Rituals in Psychotherapy – Transition and Continuity" (New York:Irvington) 1996 p. 95.

The pastoral presence should cultivate an awareness of the phase through which the person who has suffered the loss is passing The person with a pastoral heart should be alert to the need for sufficient time to be allowed for grief as well as the appropriateness for some rite which gives some closure to the grieving period. Often an unorthodox and imaginative informal rite needs to be offered to effect an appropriate healing of grief and make observers aware that their friend's grieving period is over and now is the time for normal living. Normal relationships, reactions and business can now safely be resumed.

Following a significant loss a "time to grieve" must be allowed, as well, permission to resume a full active life must be recognized. It may well be appropriate to initiate an informal or formal rite to enable the mourner to fully return to their life in the community.

CHAPTER 5

A Child's Questions About Death

Working in a major Pediatric Hospital and being daily involved with families who had a child terminally ill and subsequently died, it was possible to draw alongside the family members from toddlers to grandparents. The most seriously confused are the children ten years and younger. Thirty-five years ago, I was able to produce an illustrated booklet with the above title to put into the hands of the children or for the parents to read to the children. Funeral homes, hospital social workers and chaplains and others used it extensively. It is now out of print and the illustrations dated. The gist of most of the questions, are considered in this chapter.

The Puzzled Child – "Am I going to die?"

For a child up to the age of eight years and even ten years, death is a mystery. Perhaps during this age bracket they are encountering the death of a human for the first time. It may be an older relative, a neighbor, some one they have heard about at school or preschool. Their minds keep ticking away trying to understand what has happened and why. Somehow, their elders are silent about it, brushing any query aside or changing the subject. To tell a child that they are too young to understand compounds their dilemma and fear. This obvious avoidance of adults to include them in such conversations, keeps them ignorant and still questioning about what happened or else they are sent off to stay somewhere else until after the funeral is over. Even very young children are perceptive of change and the more somber the atmosphere at home or other familiar places, the more they are aware that something is not right. Their small minds are perplexed and sometimes are fearful that something dreadful might befall them and that their parents are trying to protect them from it or at worst plotting against them.

It becomes more relevant to them if their sibling dies. Here one day and not around the next. Perhaps, the parents may say, "your sister or brother got sick or had an accident and died." They are excluded from all other conversation. So often they are ignored and shut out, because the parents don't know how to deal with the questions.

> *When the words, 'death', 'dead', and 'died' are overheard even during the most guarded conversations the child's mental gymnastics turn over the question, "What is death."*

When the words, 'death', 'dead', and 'died' are overheard even during the most guarded conversations the child's mental gymnastics turn over the question, "What is death." The conspiracy of secrecy builds up fears and the child becomes convinced that death is sinister and that they might also die soon. Soon another question starts running around in their minds, "Am I going to die soon?"

There does not have to be a human death to raise the subject of dying with a pre-schooler or older children. Opportunities to explain death that all living things die often occur around them. If these opportunities are taken before a human death is faced many of these fears may be eliminated.

In a house or in the garden, flowers are on show. The child regularly sees flower petals fallen on the table, in the garden or on the lawn. Such is a good time to raise the question of dying. Explain that these flowers have shown their beauty and shared their perfume, giving pleasure to those who saw and smelt them. The energy to keep itself alive had run out, so they died.

Driving along a highway it is common to see an animal; or bird that has been killed by traffic. This may be explained that they were near the road and were dazzled by the headlights of a car and truck and could not get out of the way. Another explanation is to turn it into a safety lesson by indicating that the bird or animal was on the road and without carefully looking walked or flew onto the road and was hit by the bus. This may be added to, by saying that all animals die like Johnny's pet bird even Sarah's cuddly cat or dog will die someday.

When someone dies or our pet dog or cat dies, we all feel sad because we will not see them again. However we have photographs we can look at and our memories will recall all the happy times we had with the grandparent, parent, brother sister, dog, bird or cat. We cannot give them a big hug, nor they give us, but we have memories of happy times with them.

This can lead to into a statement that all living things die; from plants, to animals and humans. All that grows requires sufficient food to gain strength to grow. That strength is gained by the plant or body turning the food into sap, leaves and flowers or blood, muscle and energy. In a human, the parts of the body that change our food are our stomachs, hearts, lungs, livers, kidneys etc. These get overworked and wear out like a car's engine until there is not enough strength left to breathe and eat properly. For some, one or more of these body parts may get sick and not work so well, even when they are not so old. Today, doctors and nurses are able to give medicines to help a sick person get better. There are some sicknesses that will not let the medicine work to make them better so they die.

People, animals and plants, i.e. all things that live on earth must die at some time.

Why Do People Die?

This question moves on from what we have been talking about. Our bodies consist of working parts that wear out, just like an engine. Grandma and grandpa cannot run around and play games like a child or young person or even like they did a few years ago.

In these days people are living much longer, more are living to be over 100 years of age. This can be put down to more nutritious food, the work of doctors who are able to cure our illnesses before they do too much damage to our important organs including our brains. Others, in special cases, may live longer because when their heart, lungs or liver have difficulty in working properly they may have them replaced by what we call donor organs from someone who has just died. This process known as organ transplants keeps many thousands of people alive around the world who would have died. Depending on their age they may live for another twenty or thirty years. Eventually, people who have received a donor organ or organs die.

There are some babies born whose grandparent or parents had problem health conditions. This makes their children more likely to develop the same illnesses as they grow older. Heart weaknesses and some forms of cancer are included in these illnesses.

At times, there are what are called epidemics, which spread throughout the population. Influenza, measles and chicken pox are common epidemics and if it is a bad variety of them, they can cause death. Mosquitoes carry illnesses such as Malaria, Ross River and Dengue Fevers that are attributed to mosquito bites. Through these, people may die.

There are all sorts of other reasons why people die; including accidents of all sorts, even earthquakes, fires, hurricanes, cyclones and war.

Do only Old People Die?

A century ago, more died under the age of five years than died of old age that was then considered to be over sixty years. The anti-malarial programs and the control of cholera, typhoid, small-pox, diphtheria and other epidemics as well as improved hygiene and obstetric procedures has reduced infant and early childhood mortality world wide. Also, the use of anti-biotics has also helped reduced the number of early deaths.

A person may die at any age. The Australian Aborigine believed that to die under five years or old age was natural. To die in between was due to sorcery or the casting of spells. The tribal elders sought to find out, who the person was that cast the spell. The named sorcerer had a bone pointed at him and he died within three days. The elders' judgment and act caused the alleged sorcerer to believe he would die and he did in that time because his mind controlled his body. In modern western society, some have so much hardship and troubles that they similarly do not wish to live and so the mind takes over and they die earlier than they normally would have. Their will to live had gone.

Sometimes they die because they get so sick that the doctor cannot help them to get better. Other times they die because they have had a bad accident. Not everybody who gets sick or has an accident dies. Most sick people or people who have an accident get better after sometime of medical treatment.

There are people who become involved in accidents on land, air or in the water and are killed. These may be caused by carelessness, thoughtlessness, bad workmanship or maintenance, or inefficiency. Another major cause of death before old age is when people take their own lives in one way or another. This is called suicide.

This type of answer often is sufficient to satisfy a child. However, it should be adjusted to suit the age of the child. They will go away and think about it. If they are not satisfied they will return with another question. This new question again must be answered simply, directly and honestly. Adults often confuse the child more by going beyond the question itself. By doing this it opens the child's mind to other involved questions. In cases, where you cannot answer the question, be honest and say, "I don't know." There is a danger in making something up in order to satisfy the child. By admitting that you have no answer, the child will respect you for your honesty.

In answering this question, "Do only old people die?" the word 'sometimes' is useful. Yes, sometimes babies die when they are born. Sometimes boys and girls die. Sometimes, mummies and daddies may die. In using this, care should be taken not to instill undue fear of their own, their siblings or their parents' early death.

Remember this question is an indication of an underlying fear. Unless that fear is able to be expelled the child may develop psychological problems or phobias, such as; a fear of crossing a busy road, of going to a doctor, going to visit in a hospital, getting in a car after a serious accident, etc. Pastoral responsibility recognizes the seriousness of this question.

Death Makes Me Scared?

When someone has died adults often discuss what happened. That children are in the room is often ignored. The adults talk in language well above the ability of the child to understand. They hear conversations like; "It's a blessing she died. He was in pain and had suffered a lot. The wounds she received were horrifying. I don't know how he lasted so long. The family should have called the doctor earlier and she might still be with us. I don't think the Doctor knew what he was doing. The hospital did their best but it was hopeless from the start. Poor Lucy, I don't know how she will manage without him; she will be lost. She depended upon him so much."

A young child hearing this type of talk uses a child's vivid imagination to conjure up all sorts of dreadful scenes. His imagination knows no limit because he has seen some of the most horrendous scenes on television and in video-games where violence and death are savagely enacted. The worse of these screen depictions are applied to the person who had died and is thought to be what is being talked about by the adults in the room.

When a parent or other trusted adult is alone with a child, the child may remark, "Death makes me scared." For a child, death is a scary thing to talk about. There are few people who can satisfactorily talk to a child about death. Children sometimes discuss among themselves their concepts of death which are often unrealistic and can be further frightening for a child.

It is best to admit right from the beginning to answer this question frankly and say;

"Yes, we can often feel afraid when we hear talk about death or about a person who has died. This is because we don't really understand all about it, not even adults. We feel sad and unhappy when someone has died because we will never anymore see that person at home, at school, at church, at the park, or anywhere else where we used to see them. I don't really know where they have gone or what it is like to be dead because I have never died nor been there myself. (Notice the use of the first person in that last sentence. It puts the child more on your level.). When we don't know everything about something we often try to imagine the worst."

"When you feel scared about death, try to think of something good about death such as the person will never again be hurt or feel pain and will never get sick again. They will never be involved in an accident again or have broken legs or arms. Just fancy never having to cry."

Positive thoughts, sown into a child's thinking while not providing an answer to all their queries about fearing death, will help to relieve them of some negative images.

Do People Feel Death?

To a young child, death is often a bigger mystery because all the pictures of death they see are of a body or bodies lying on the ground. Little minds are constantly exploring, discovering, and trying to understand the big wild world in which they live. When they hear that someone has died their minds go into vivid action recall as they think about it. They try to image what it would be like to be dead. Hence, comes this very realistic question, "Do people feel death?"

It may be approached something like this: "If you fall over and skin your knee, what part of your body hurts? (The child will reply that it is the knee.) If you hit your head on the open cupboard door, where does it feel sore? (The child replies, 'Where I bumped it.') How do you know that your knee or your head hurt? It may be explained to the child that the body has messengers that run back to the brain and tells it where it hurts. These messengers are called nerves. The nerves or messengers are kept active and alert when our mind is working well. When death comes our spirits leave our body and the nerves stop working. If the messengers are not working the body cannot feel any pain."

"There are times, when the messengers shut down because we are very ill, unconscious, or our head has had a big blow, or a doctor has given us an injection or medicine to put the nerves to sleep. It is like being in a deep sleep and again the body feels nothing. That is why doctors can operate on a person in hospital and they do not feel what the doctor is doing. In death, we feel nothing because these messengers cannot work.

The child needs to be reassured that no pain is felt. Sometimes, a child may think that their deceased grandmother may be feeling pain in death. Such a thought can severely disturb a child in many ways, especially during their sleep. This is an important question which if left unanswered can lead to a much stressed out child.

Why Don't All People in Hospital Get Better?

There are few children growing up that do not pass a hospital a number of times. They will also hear ambulances with sirens screaming taking people to hospital. They see ambulances at accident sites preparing to take the injured to hospital.

> *In death, we feel nothing because these messengers cannot work.*

These same children will hear of doctors and nurses in hospitals working to help sick and injured people to get well. Perhaps some of their play friends have been taken to hospital and have returned to play as hard as they used to do.

Maybe they know of an adult or relative who had a stay in a hospital and went home again. They may remember when their mother went to hospital and came home with their baby brother or sister and both were well. Then a relative, family friend or someone from the neighborhood was rushed to hospital and never came home again. The person had died.

The child is bewildered. They have known several people go to hospital and come home again. Now this other person does not. It is natural for the child to ask, "Why don't all people in hospital get better?"

At the back of such a question is a rising fear that hospitals may not be a safe place to go. You might never come out again. It is necessary that any fear of hospitals should be squashed as early as possible. The focus should be on the hospital helping people to get better.

It should be emphasized with the child: "Hospitals with their doctors and nurses do try their best to make people well. Some are sick and by an operation or taking special medicine or other treatment, they are able to go home and live a normal life. Other people are very very sick, neither medicine nor operations are able to cure them so the doctors are able to give them medicine that will ease any pain or discomfort and make them comfortable. Knowing that they will die, the doctors make it as restful as possible for them. A hospital is a good place to go when you are sick."

Do Only Naughty People Die?

A child may hear of accidents where through a child's carelessness or thoughtlessness a child is killed. This may be when a child runs across the road chasing a ball and is hit by a car. A toddler may have fallen into the home swimming pool and drowned when they were told not to go near the pool. Another child may have been playing with matches setting his clothes on fire causing severe burns to his body which caused his death

Parents on hearing of such cases may say to their children, "See what happens when you are naughty; and run on the road, go near the pool without mummy or daddy present or play with matches." Those words sink in so death becomes associated with naughtiness. So, if they hear of a person or a child dying they wonder what they did wrong to deserve to die. A sensitive child can become fearful when they have done something wrong. They may even hide to escape the punishment of death or remain silent and tense waiting for something to happen. The above cases may be the only types of death they have heard about so they are likely to ask the question, "Do only naughty people die?"

It is a very serious question, Just to laugh it off as say, "Of course not!" may cause further tension for the child because their important question seemed not to be taken seriously. Children see laughter in such situations as derision and scorn which can be damaging to the child who may not pursue the question further and retain the apprehensions that they have been harboring. Any opportunity to help the child understand may have been lost, causing the child to withdraw from activity to avoid being naughty and therefore not die.

It needs to be carefully explained to the child that all people die. Death is not a punishment for being naughty or being sinful. In accidents, it is often a case of being in the wrong place at the wrong time. It is not God or anyone else punishing people for being naughty.

It may be pointed out that when born, it was in God's mind that we should all live a normal life until we were at least seventy years of age. That was God's plan. When we don't look after our bodies, catch a germ, don't eat properly, work too hard without sufficient rest or do things that are risky or dangerous we may die younger than our seventy years. Some people die early because they smoke cigarettes, take drugs, or drink a lot of alcohol. These all do damage to our body such as our heart, lungs, liver and brain.

No one dies an early death because God is angry with them and certainly not as a punishment for being naughty.

Can I Wish a Person to Death?

This is one of the most serious questions that may be encountered when dealing with children and death. Several times I have come across it or the effects of this question being ignored.

As a child, sometimes a brother, sister or playmates do something hurtful to a child. A parent may refuse to permit their child to do something, go somewhere or give them something. The child gets angry and boils inside and then in a spiteful rage says, "I wish you were dead." Perhaps we can all recall times when as a child we have thought or actually said those words, to a sibling or even our mother or father when we have not got our own way.

For the multitude of times that thought is expressed or repressed nothing ever happens. On the odd occasion shortly after the words enter the mind the person against whom those words applied got sick and died or was killed in an accident. The child immediately thinks that the person died because they wished them dead. As a result, the child is filled with guilt and sometimes with a sense of fear and terror at the possibility of punishment for their death wish. After the death of the person against whom the death wish was made, the child may become abnormally quiet and want to be alone. It may be more than the normal grief reaction. Extra sensitive attention should be paid to such a child.

> *Our wishes cannot cause death. Our thoughts are not that powerful.*

That attention should try to draw the child out by talking about the nature of the death; if it was an illness then the nature of the onset should be described; if it was an accident then the cause of the accident is able to be explained; if anyone else is involved in the accident then their role in the accident should be spelled out to show the child was not involved.

When the child openly admits to uttering the death wish the opportunity should then be taken to point out that our wishes cannot cause death. Our thoughts are not that powerful. The nature of the death should once more be stressed as not being caused by what the child or anyone else said against the deceased.

It will take time for the child to be convinced it is not his or her fault. It is possible that these guilt feelings will occasionally recur many months after the event. Any unusual behavior of the child should be continually monitored.

It is not Fair

This isn't so much a question, as a statement about the child's true feelings about the death of a loved person or pet. To put it in adult language, it means, "Why is life so unfair to me?"

As the child is growing up, security and love of certain people are very important. If one or more of these special people die they feel they have been robbed. Some children may get hysterical screaming and crying; but unlike a toy they smashed in a hysterical tantrum, this is more serious, the loved person cannot be replaced.   If it is a much loved grandparent, aunt, mother, father, or sibling, the child knows they will never see them again. Their sense of loss is intense. It is not unnatural to hear the child stamp their feet as they cry out, "It isn't fair." Whether the person is old or young, it just, is not fair. It is indeed unfair, when as a child, one you love has died and left you. They had and would have continued to play an important, helpful and loving part in the child's life.

No one dies an early death because God is angry with them and certainly not as a punishment for being naughty.

The child may be helped to understand that there are many boys and girls who lose someone who is very close to them. At that very moment there are thousands also feeling the same way that it isn't fair. Initially, it is essential to support the child in the sense of unfairness, to do otherwise would be to alienate the child's response to you.

Gradually, you may be able to talk about the good things that the deceased did for the child. The more you can get the child to talk about the deceased the better. The occasional interjection like, "You were lucky to have such a good friend/grandma all these years." The occasional interjection may be able to be turned around to saying, "You have a lot to be thankful for."

The idea of getting the child to say, 'thank you' for the person's love and care is a step forward. It also may be gently pointed out that their life would not have been so happy if they had never known the person who had died. From there, the conversation may lead onto all the people he or she has around her who still love and care for him or her and that they will meet other new people who will also be able to give help and support. The aim is to get the child to appreciate those she has who still love her. A child at this stage is still hurting and these moves must be taken very slowly and not hurried.

> *We believe heaven is a place where God is. Because God is love, heaven will be a place full of love.*

It is difficult to minister to a grieving child at this stage and it requires special inspiration that is best obtained through allowing the Holy Spirit to give the appropriate words each time you open your mouth.

Is the Dead Person Sleeping?

It may be explained to a child that when we are asleep our minds and our bodies are resting. Because we are not moving and using our legs and arms our heart doesn't have to pump so hard, so, it is getting a little rest. Sleep gives us strength for another day at school or play. Sleep is necessary if we are to remain healthy and happy.

When a person dies the body stops working. Their lungs stop breathing and their hearts stop pumping and so everything else stops working. Sleep and death are very different. In sleep, we wake up; in death, we do not.

What Happens to Dead People?

This is a common question that children ask. If they do not ask it, they think about it and just wonder. A house can be a good starting point.

We live in a house. The people living inside it make it a home. Our bodies are like a home, we have a spirit which lives inside our body to make it a home.

When a person dies, the body becomes an empty house. Most people believe that the spirit which made the body a home has left and gone to heaven. Our spirit lives in, but does not die like the rest of the body. It is with our spirit that we are able to love and receive love. The body of a dead person cannot love or receive love.

The spirit or soul never wears out. We cannot see someone's spirit, nor can we see heaven. We believe that we have a spirit and that there is a heaven. This is what we call faith. Faith is something we can not fully understand yet accept it as being true. Peoples of all religions believe that we have a spirit which lives in our bodies and leaves us when we die.

What Is Heaven Like?

This question is one that all people ask openly or question within themselves. Toward the end of life it becomes more relevant

A child may be told: "We don't know what heaven looks like. We cannot tell you where it is. We know that our bodies wear out, get ill, or we are involved in an accident and die. Because it is our spirit alone that lives on, we believe that we shall not again experience the sadness, the trouble and the difficulties we had on earth.

We believe heaven is a place where God is. Because God is love, heaven will be a place full of love. We need not be fearful about heaven. Therefore we can look forward to happiness, love and peace in heaven." Paul, in the Christian's New Testament, tells us than when we die we are given a new spiritual body that is not like our earthly body. It has no bones, hearts and lungs etc. because our spirit does not need them after our bodies die. In our new spiritual body we go to join the people who have died before us. We cannot describe this place because we haven't seen it and cannot see pictures of it.

What Is a Funeral?

Children hear about funerals. It is announced in church. That so and so's funeral will be held next Wednesday. They see a Funeral Home's hearse with a casket in the back. On television, funerals often are seen on the screen both on the news and in sit-coms. So children have mental pictures of funerals.

A child may be told that a funeral is a special time spent remembering and saying goodbye to a dead person. The body of the person is placed in a box which is called a casket or coffin.

Those who loved and respected the dead person meet at the funeral to share their feelings of love for the person. They talk about the good and the not so good things about the dead one which helps to take away some of the sadness.

There is often much crying at the funeral. The crying shows how much the person who died was liked and loved and how much they cared. Not everybody cries. It is okay to cry and it okay not to cry at a funeral. The important thing, the funeral gives us is the opportunity to express our feelings of sadness at not being able to again have earthly fellowship with the deceased again.

What Happens to Our Bodies When We Die?

Children see cemeteries and may hear about crematoria but do not fully understand what they are all about.

After the funeral service, the casket in which the body is, is lowered into the ground at the cemetery which is the place where the bodies of dead people are buried. This is called the grave site. At the grave site, usually a head stone, cross or some other erection is made with the person's name and details. Sometimes it is a family plot and several members of the family are buried in the same area. Family members sometimes bring fresh flowers and place them on the grave or may even make a little garden and grow some small attractive plants. In the grave the body turns into soil like all dead things.

Other bodies are taken to a place called a Crematorium where the body is more quickly turned into ashes. It is a place where there are lots of flowers and trees. Each plant has a name in front of it reminding relatives and friends that this is where their family member's ashes were placed. Other people's ashes are placed in a small hole in a brick wall, called a niche, with the name of the person on a brass plate. In some cases, the relatives take the ashes and sprinkle them over a place especially loved by the family.

In the cemetery or the crematorium the body feels no pain because the spirit, which is the important part of us, has already gone to heaven.

How Can I Stop Feeling sad?

A child's pet dog or cat has died; the child's grandmother or other relative or family friend has died and they feel sad for a long time after the death. The child sometimes may ask, "How may I stop feeling sad." It is an important question for them and needs answering.

When someone we love dies, it is like when we cut our finger peeling an apple. It hurts very much even after putting on some ointment and bandaging it. When someone had died, a child may feel angry as well as sad about it. Some may even feel like hating the person for going away and making them feel so hurt and sad. They may even call God nasty names for letting the person die.

> *When someone we love dies, it is like when we cut our finger peeling an*

It will be helpful for them to talk to someone they can trust about how they feel. When another person listens to you it helps. Let them cry if they feel like it and be sad. They do not have to cry if they do not want to. Like the cut finger the soreness and pain will get less and less when they start to do the things they used to do and play with their friends.

Am I Going to Die Too?

The unknown about death keeps the child's imaginative mind working. It is inevitable that they will start wondering if and when they are going to die. The question, "Am I going to die, too," goes through their minds. It is often a question that may be asked as they are being tucked into bed at night. The question should be dealt with then or else it may trouble their minds and disturb their sleep.

God really wanted all of us to live until we grow old, i.e. when our aged bodies find it too hard to keep going. There are some babies who die when they are born because they were very sick. We can die at any age because of a bad illness or an accident. We should expect to live a long time because doctors, today, can do many wonderful things when we are sick and even when we are hurt in an accident.

We all should live each day as if we are going to live until we are old. It is only the unusual that causes us to die earlier. At their age they should be encouraged and assured when they go to sleep and not to be afraid that they will not wake up in the morning.

Did God Make My Brother or Sister Die?

At a funeral service and around the time of a death a child may hear the name of God a number of times. So God and death become jumbled in the mind of the child. The child may think God has something to do with the death. Some parents may make that link with the child when they don't know how else to answer the child's question about death.

Some outrageous explanations have been made by relatives and church people to children in response to a child's questions. God loved your little brother so much that he took him to be with Him. God wanted another little angel in Heaven so he picked your little sister and now she is flying around with the other boy and girl angels.

> *"Am I going to die, too," goes through their minds. It is often a question that may be asked as they are being tucked into bed at night.*

These are two of the type of responses I have heard people say to children. God is virtually being blamed for the death of a sibling or other loved one. God may be seen as selfish for wanting their sibling with Him.

Many a practicing atheist has been driven to such a hatred of a feelingless, selfish God, so that as they grew older they jettison all concept of the existence of a God. Alternatively, some people are anti-god and anti-church because they cannot accept or believe in a cruel God who would willfully take away a sibling, parent or grandparent from a child. Such glib answers shift the blame of the death onto God and are often very damaging to the ultimate spiritual life of the child A simple answer often suffices a young child

God or Jesus did not cause your sister or brother to die. God's plan was that people should live to about the age of seventy years or more. That is a long time. God meant us to live until we had children and grandchildren and be happy. Sometimes sickness and bugs cause us to get very sick and die. Sometimes other people are selfish, careless or thoughtless and cause accidents or spread their disease. Other people often die because other people do the wrong thing.

> *We all should live each day as if we are going to live until we are old.*

God never does wrong. God doesn't cause people to die.

Do Mummy and Daddy Really Love Me?

In dealing with families of Oncology patients in a children's hospital, I found, this was a question that many of the families of a patient had to face.

For example, a leukemia child can spend the major part of a year in hospital. This requires the mother or other family members to stay close by in a place like Ronald MacDonald House near the Hospital. The whole of the family life is seriously disrupted. The mother is not around for the other children before and after school. Sometimes they don't see her all week. Dad is not as good a cook as mum is. Dad is often at the hospital at the weekends while mum is at home catching up, so they can't take the children to sports, other parents have to do it. Family finances are hard hit with medical expenses, travel costs and the extra costs of living away from home. The budget has to be restricted so that the brother may have to forego a school excursion and the other siblings forgo many of their usual things. The other family members are suffering, one or two may have been wondering, why their parents spend so much time and money on the sick child and neglect them. "Perhaps, mother and father don't love me as much as the one who is sick!" This is a situation that must be dealt with. Any failure to do so may result in a brood of resentful, rebellious teenagers, a few years later.

A satisfactory explanation is necessary such as: "When a family member is sick and dying there is need for either mummy or daddy to be at the hospital most of the time. The doctors and nurses try to make your sick brother well. Sometimes they need the help of your mother or father. Your brother is very sick and gets very frightened at what is happening to him. Without his mother or father with him much of the time, he would be much worse. He needs to see that the whole family love him and care for him. If you were in his position they would do the same for you. They love you equally as much but your brother has a special need of us at the present time. If he gets better they will make it up to you. If he does not live then you will be getting a lot more attention for a long time.

The Church and Children's Questions.

The church should be aware of some of these questions which are often faced when a young family experiences a significant death. A person who has the ability to get alongside children and speak using words that the children understand, should be alerted to the possibility of such questions arising and be deputed to ascertain if the children are having any problems such as these.

It is better for these or similar approaches such as these be presented to the children in a logical and constructive way rather than some of the outrageous, frightening and damaging explanations given by some not so knowledgeable, well-meaning, Christians. Properly handled, an encounter with death by a child can be turned into a practical learning experience about life and make God's love more relevant to them.

CHAPTER 6

The Diagnosis is Cancer

For more than ten years, one of my allocations was to the Hematology Unit of a major Teaching Hospital involved in cooperative research with international programs. The Hematology ward deals with those suffering from cancer and other related blood diseases. I usually saw each patient daily from the day of diagnosis. Every patient reacts differently to the doctor's pronouncement and also to the treatment. Each patient needed an empathetic listening ear or just the presence of a person not wearing a doctor's coat or a nurse's uniform. Some would be so shocked that any word about religion from a chaplain would be an intrusion. For someone just to sit and hold the patient's hand was the most consoling presence possible. Others may be talkative about all the tasks that they have not finished and cannot afford the time to be in hospital. Their minds might again be full of concerns for their loved ones and how would they manage without them. At another bedside, the chaplain may have to listen to a non-stop tirade against the injustices of the world, life and God or be so quiet and timid in fear of the prospects of an early death or be emotionally distraught as they thought about how a premature death would affect all their plans. In these early days after diagnosis, it was necessary to let the patient be able to react according to their personality and circumstances. By letting them, reveal their feelings it was easier to be able to understand them and the best way to get alongside them in a meaningful relationship.

Ignorance.

To mention the word 'cancer' to a patient is like confronting the patient with an obnoxious ogre. For most people it sounds as if the death knell is tolling. Ignorance concerning cancer in the community is rife. Cancer is one of the most feared words in the dictionary. It has terrifying connotations which arose a century ago when all cancers were incurable. Most people see it as the worst type of death possible – an agonizing death with the wasting away of the body. In modern times when further helpful treatment for the cancer is impossible, pain, is able to be relieved with palliative medication. There are few properly managed people who should be suffering unbelievable pain. It should be remembered that in this 21st. century a large percentage of cancer is curable and other patients are able to go into remission for years.

For the average, newly diagnosed cancer patient, their ignorance of the cancer, its type, treatment and outcomes make their condition frightening and unbelievable. They can only remember anecdotal accounts of cancer patients who suffered much and who lost all their hair. Fear and panic often overwhelms them which are not helped by their family's pessimistic and perhaps hysterical reactions. Death and incurability are two words the average person associates with the word.

The Patient's Early Reactions

A person is not feeling well, so they go to the doctor to ascertain the problem in order to be treated and resume normal activities in a few days or weeks at the most. Few would seriously suspect cancer unless there was a family history of cancer. For the unsuspecting patient there are five major emotional reactions to the diagnosis.

- Fear
- Anger
- Hopelessness
- Desperation
- Insecurity

Fear

The first reaction is naturally fear generated by the word 'cancer'. It is publicly presumed that death by cancer is the worst possible way to die. There are other medical conditions which in my opinion are far less desirable. Those involving neurological function may be much more inhospitable. In the minds of many, the mention of the word, 'cancer', spells out the word "DEATH".

Death has the air of finality about it. The mind is preoccupied with trying to come to grips with those two words death and cancer. They seem synonymous. As the prognosis sinks in, the familiar sights and objects of beauty are looked upon with a sense of impending loss. The repeated inner response to those eye and mind enriching sights is, "Not much longer." For some it may be the last time they will see them and enjoy their pleasure. All around them they are reminded of the impending finality to all earthly things for them.

For a young person in their teens or early adulthood, the diagnosis destroys their dreams of love, marriage, family, career prospects, academic achievements, sporting and other aspirations. There is a looming finality to all these. Even for older people the idea of growing old gracefully and in happy comfortable retirement has been dealt a sickening blow. Their mental reveries about the future have been exchanged for fear of pain, hospitals, uncertain physical mobility and loss of everything considered of value and worth, including relationships. For What? - An unknown mysterious future life. The fear of the unknown helps to accentuate the fear of the impending perceived ravages of an inhumane disease with its pain and indignation. Fear stalks the mind. Fear conjures up horrifying images. Fear leaves the patient with the desire to curl up in a fetal position in the hope much of the physical torment will pass over them.

> *Death has the air of finality about it. The mind is preoccupied with trying to come to grips with those two words death and cancer.*

Anger

All shattering of future prospects by the pronouncement of cancer stirs up a deep seated anger, There will be those whose spiritual communication with God enables them to accept what lies before them and will maintain a confidence that the one to whom they have committed their lives will provide the necessary comfort, and strength to cope with whatever there is to be experienced.

For many there wells up a deep bitterness and resentment toward the same God who has allowed their condition to develop. They blame God for it all. They try to justify their anger by protesting that they have lived a good and just life and do not deserve it. They even may claim that they have never deliberately hurt either man or animal. The infliction of cancer upon them is totally unjustified. This anger may cause them to be uncooperative, sullen and belligerent toward all including medical and nursing staff. Some days, this is more evident than others. A pastoral person must be prepared to accept any vitriolic accusations against God, the Church and themselves as a representative of the church. Acceptance of such tirades without any attempts to defend or exonerate God or the church will do much to quell the deep-seated venom.

> *For many there wells up a deep bitterness and resentment toward the same God who has allowed their condition to develop.*

It has been my experience that by careful and sensitive handling these very angry people ultimately welcome pastoral support.

Hopelessness

Cancer has retained the popularly conceived notion that it inflicts a hopeless situation. This, no doubt, persists because of all the different organizations that regularly make public appeals for research to cure cancer. A sense of hopelessness affects some cancer patients so much that they have no fighting spirit or determination to beat the disease.

It is encouraging to see women who have survived breast cancer to be publicly encouraging their stricken sisters with evidence that their cancer is not necessarily a knock out blow, and that many cases of cancer are curable if caught and treated in time.

For so many, the diagnosis leads them to see only the worst prognosis, which is all that their angry, fearful minds can soak up. This feeling of hopelessness may take over the throne of their thinking ousting anger and fear from the centre of the court. "It is all hopeless what is the use of trying to combat it; may as well curl up and die; why persist with the treatment when it won't work" are some of the thoughts that run through their mind as they take their chemotherapy or sit in radiology. "It's all of no use; treatment only prolongs the agony; there is no way of escaping its clutches" are further seductive thoughts rising from this ruling sense of hopelessness. They might even pray to God to let them die quickly and to get it all over and finished.

> *In this age of information technology, the internet is one of the first sources resorted to.*

Desperation

This sense of despair can lead them to desperation. Many in trying to dispel this sense of hopelessness will, in desperation, clutch at anything to avoid the painful development of cancer's grip and give them some hopeful anticipation. A cancer diagnosis will scatter friends and relatives in all directions seeking anecdotal success stories of others who have experienced some relief from cancer. The fact, that each person's cancer is different, and each person's body metabolism and immune systems vary widely are never considered. So and so, by using this or that treatment overcame their cancer is the only criteria needing consideration to try the same treatment.

In this age of information technology, the internet is one of the first sources resorted to. No matter what the subject, you can get numerous articles related to the topic. There are articles offered by specialists, pseudo-specialists and non-specialists with a very diverse range of conclusions and often, only presumed success or otherwise concerning cancer and its treatment. This information taken collectively will appear contradictory when it comes to particular treatments and their success and failures. Whether it is the patients or relatives and friends, their choice of material to accept and follow will be selective and subjective. This selectivity is biased toward successful results and if followed, may produce false hopes if they abandon the oncologist's treatment entirely and take up some other type of therapy. To accept and follow any regimen without full awareness of the authenticity, qualifications and dependability of the source is unwise.

Medical science offers three conventional treatments depending on the type, nature and stage of the cancer's development. This is typical of American, European and Australian treatment which specializes in surgery, chemotherapy and radiation according to the cancer, its stage of development and the overall physical and medical condition of the patient. The purpose of chemotherapy and radiation is to shrink the tumor and if possible, eradicate it or enable surgery to be performed. These often produce unpleasant side effects which may include severe nausea and hair loss thus further temporarily reducing the patient's quality of life.

However, there are some treatments which may be considered as complementary. They are able to assist conventional medicine in bringing about a remission. The function of complementary therapies should be to boost the immune system so that the T cells or cancer killing cells can function more efficiently and quickly. These complimentary treatments may include some Chinese medicine such as: acupuncture, herbal and naturopathic medicine, massage, nutrition, yoga, meditation and other relaxation techniques. Such treatments may benefit the immune system and relax the mind.

Natural Therapies. Therapies that offer a nutritious diet, build up the body and help in countering the toxic effects of chemotherapy and radiation. Conventional therapies stress the body and break down the immune system leaving them more open to infections. A well nourished body improves metabolic function. Cancer is considered a metabolic disease. Metabolism is the sum of the processes or chemical changes in an organism or cell by which food is built up into living protoplasm and by which protoplasm is broken down into simpler compounds with the exchange of energy.

Meditation and relaxation. These are religious in origin and content. They relax tension, improving immune functions, which are able to make the treatment more effective. Relaxation minimizes many of the negative effects of some of the reactions to the diagnosis which affect the body chemistry. Stress can hasten the cancer's growth and reduce the effectiveness of any treatment. Meditation and the calling upon spiritual resources have a significant complementary role alongside the treatment. Relaxation aids the mind to let go of the negative emotions and helps fulfill the need to affirm the positive aspects and future possibilities.

Enhanced immune responses and relaxed minds are able to more harmoniously assist in producing more positive results for the conventional treatments leading to less discomfort, remission and in some cases cure.

If complementary treatment is being considered or practiced, the patient should be warned to carefully check the credentials of the other therapist and be aware of the side effects of the treatment and its compatibility with the oncologist's medicinal protocol. The oncologist and the local general practitioner should be kept informed of the nature of the herbal or other medications being prescribed by a complementary therapist.

The desperate search for a cure or a quick fix via complementary medicine should be, with caution, researched and reliably evaluated before any hasty, desperate commitment, on anecdotal or unsubstantiated and non-researched recommendations from other unauthenticated sources, are made.

Desperation may drive any cancer patient to a faith or so-called spiritual healer for a miraculous cure. I have encountered several who have taken this course. They have told me how they have had hands laid on them, prayed over and been cured. In most cases these have carried a self-confident, arrogant attitude back to the hospital and its staff. One such woman at a very critical stage was to have a bone marrow transplant boasted, "I don't need this bone-marrow transplant, I've been cured." She died in Intensive Care three weeks later.

> *Faith healers are often show-men out to boost their own egos and seldom in the practice of their daily lives give God any glory.*

Faith healers are often show-men out to boost their own egos and seldom in the practice of their daily lives give God any glory. Many of their so-called healings are case of mind over matter until the psychological euphoria has died down. I have seen crutches left down the front of the church as the person started to walk back to their seat with much joyful applause, only to collapse half-way back up the aisle on their way to their seat. On occasions, usually in more reserved situations with people who are genuinely spiritually in tune with God a miraculous cure may be possible.

Desperation efforts to find a cure often create further distress of mind and confusion making response to conventional treatment all the more difficult. Faith in a possible cure when unrealized may incur deeper depressive reactions or guilt at not being worthy of a cure. Such failed efforts may throw the patient into greater state of despondency, further risking the opportunity for the treatment to succeed.

Insecurity

Cancer drives home our sense of vulnerability and human frailties. The business executive, the building laborer, the medical doctor, the shop assistant, the school teacher or the unemployed may be found in the same oncology unit undergoing chemotherapy or radiation for cancer. Wealth or lack of wealth, status or absence of status, educated or illiterate, skilled or unskilled, it makes no difference. Anyone may or may not be diagnosed with cancer. Cancer is no respecter of persons or their social profile.

Cancer means we are not in control of our bodies nor of their functions. It puts us into the hands of others whose decisions will physically and materially affect our future. Others direct our treatment; others dictate our periods in hospital; others tell us what we should or should not do. The feeling of insecurity is one of the strongest emotions, which also has a bearing upon the physical condition. This insecurity results from the inability to make decisions or to determine what is going to happen, even, to our family and loved ones. The necessary confinement caused by the illness often means unemployment. Unemployment shouts 'loss of income and lifestyle for the family.' For most cancer sufferers, the illness affects a much wider circle including members of the family, fellow employees, employers and participants in the patient's other social involvements and the patient can do nothing about it. They are impotent to do anything about any thing except be obedient to the medical experts. The future is very overcast and very doubtful and out of the patient's hand to direct. To lie in bed day after day, being constantly reminded of how useless they are and all too frequently being nauseous, magnifies and further troubles the mind as to the depth of their sense of security. Nothing is certain. Nothing can be relied upon. Nothing can be predicted with confidence.

The Patient and the Doctor

An important factor, in a patient's response to the disease, is the doctor/patient relationship. This is a two-way street. The doctor must see and treat the patient as a person and not as a statistic. The patient needs to feel that he or she is not just a part moving along a production line where nimble fingers take it, fitting it, and adjusting it, and then sending it on in the inevitable process. Unless the doctor is able to add the personal touch and interest in the patient's social background and support, the patient feels like a minnow in the hands of a professional who looks down upon the patient.

In the Hematology clinical team with which I was involved, every member knew the family back-ground and who were the principle care-givers to the patient. We saw those family members had the support they required and were fully informed of the relevant updates in procedures.

The patient who feels warmth beyond the professional role is able to have a greater confidence in the words of advice and the treatment offered. The patient feels no intimidation and has a freedom to ask the specialist those deeper anxiety-producing questions. The confidence is maintained, even when a straight forward honest answer is "I don't know", or "I cannot tell you.

This team approach was abundantly evident in the clinical meetings. They showed discernment of the emotional and spiritual needs as well as the patient's support network. Another team in a pediatric oncology unit would observe with whom the child was building a deeper rapport. If a member of the domestic staff was able to get the child to respond more than others that staff member was encouraged to spend more time with the child. With other children, it may be the medical intern, a nurse, the social worker, the dietician or the chaplain. Patients must have confidence in the doctor and his or her team's professionalism and this is more firmly gained in the team's ability to understand the patient's personal needs - whether physical, social, spiritual or relationship problems. Confidence in the house doctors as well as the specialist is important if treatment is to have some positive effects, even if a cure is not possible.

> *The confidence is maintained, even when a straight forward honest answer is "I don't know", or "I cannot tell you.*

If there is any reasoned uncomfortableness with or insensitivity by the doctor, then a second opinion and association with another doctor should be considered. An unwillingness to accept a terminal diagnosis is not a reason to change the specialist. However, the patient needs to have full trust and confidence in the physician or surgeon. With such trust comes a quietening of the inner spirit which not only reduces tension and stress but is also conducive to healing and responsive to treatment. The mind often becomes ill at ease in coping with the illness and the treatment.

To newly diagnosed patients, I would stress that 50% of their bodies response to the treatment is in the mind. I have repeatedly seen this proved. In cases where the doctor's prognosis is that the patient should enter remission after the first cycle of chemotherapy, some of those whose mind could not adjust to the thought of having cancer were dead within six months. In other cases where the clinical meeting assessments were a possible six month survival at the most, where the mind was positive, they are still alive twenty-five years later.

> *A doctor must be honest in the revealing of the facts of the diagnosis and treatment protocol*

The mental approach of the patient to their illness either minimized or maximized the effectiveness of the treatment.

Mind and spirit

Norman Vincent Peale's, "Power of Positive Thinking", in the 1950's influenced not only the worlds of Psychology and Theology but also Medicine where the connection between body and mind were increasingly being identified. Since then, studies on the body, mind and medicine have been able to show the effect that positive and optimistic attitudes, including, humor and hope, play on the body's chemistry and immune systems. How a person thinks and feels affects the response to and the effectiveness of the treatment. A doctor must be honest in the revealing of the facts of the diagnosis and treatment protocol. The worst scenario as well as leaving room for some hope must be presented. To overstate the latter may very well bring about complacency, apathy, recklessness and even disregard the nature of the disease, and the need for the treatment to be taken seriously. On being given the verdict revealed by the test results of the presence of cancer, it becomes an imperative to strictly follow treatment procedures. The natural 'not me' denial reaction tends to focus upon the hope aspect and therefore minimize the seriousness of the condition. Such an action is a negative positive. In such cases, hope is stirred which is good but it often develops into an unrealistic optimism without valid foundation which is negative. It is shallow and a non-productive failure to accept the seriousness of the condition and for the treatment to be followed with due diligence. When the side effects of the treatment are starting to be felt there is a throwing up of the hands in despair and dread. Thus the cancer is able to make more rapid development due to the effect of the mind on the body's chemistry and the immune system and its ability to derive the optimum benefits from the medication or radiotherapy. The patient must be encouraged to think and determine that they may have a chance with the treatment to beat the disease.

The Pastoral Response to Cancer

We have outlined some of the early emotions stimulated by the diagnosis of cancer. The importance of the mental attitude of the cancer patient toward the doctor and the treatment has been highlighted. The person offering pastoral support to the patient and the grieving family also is integral to the patient's mental and physical response to all that is happening. Perhaps, the most significant part of the body is the spirit. The body, its organs including brain and intellectual function will in time cease to be. This body will decay and become dust or be burnt and turned into dust-like ashes. The spirit is that part of the human being which is eternal and will not die nor become dust. Therefore, we must consider the place of the spirit and cancer.

The human spirit has the capacity to be in communication with the architect of the human body - God. Through that connection, the human spirit is of divine origin and is able to make an incredible difference to the body and mind's reaction to cancer.

Some of the most unforgettable characters I have encountered, in sixty years of dealing with and pastorally caring for people, have been some cancer patients whose spirit has been in tune with God. Not once did I hear from them a word of complaint about their illness. Their faces radiated the peace and inner assurance of divine care that infected the whole unit whenever they were in for treatment. Some people will be horrified and disbelieving when I mention one of the most outstanding, was a gay man whose leukemia was a side effect from HIV/Aids.

His relationship with God was undeniable. His confidence of an early entry into God's presence was his testimony around the ward. When he was able to walk, he would each day visit each one of the more than twenty patients. In the ward, he encouraged them and shared his faith and the source of his confidence. Each life in that ward was spiritually blessed by that patient who was in his forties.

His funeral was one of the most moving that I have conducted. Spouses of deceased former patients, patients and the relatives of patients paid tribute by their presence to the spiritual blessings that flowed from him into their lives. As Jesus indicated that we shall recognize God's people by the fruit of their lives. He was a cancer patient pastorally and fruitfully ministering to other cancer patients.

Pastoral care has a role and a place in the lives of cancer sufferers who recognize and accept the possibilities of its contribution to their lives.

The Pastoral Carer and Death

I have lectured students at several tertiary institutions on "Death Education." They were professional trainees whose case loads would bring them face to face with the dying and death. These mature age students included seminarians, Government Youth Department officers, Emergency Services personnel, social workers and others. One morning during each course, they were taken to the City Morgue that had refrigeration capacity for 250 bodies holding up to 220 cadavers at any one time. It also had the capacity to perform 16 autopsies at a time. More than 90% of the students had never seen a dead body and a body undergoing an autopsy was something entirely foreign to their previous experiences. Many were shocked and aghast at what they saw. The odd person was nauseas. At the time, some thought the exercise was too harsh. Each of these students would in the future through their work be faced with death in any of its forms including mutilated accident or natural disaster bodies. Each visit was immediately followed by a debriefing session... The students were encouraged to talk about their reactions and what troubled them. At the end of the course the students considered their morgue visit one of their most helpful and positive experiences.

The purpose of the exercise was to bring these students face to face with the death of others and thereby contemplate their feelings about their own death.

Unless a person who is ministering to the dying is comfortable with their own dying and their readiness to face their own death, then their effectiveness to minister to cancer patients may be lessened, because they are unable to enter into the experience of the patient.

The Carer's Ability to Relate to the Patient

Earlier, we considered some of the emotional reactions to the news of a cancer diagnosis. Notice the terms of the popularized five stages of grief have not been used namely: shock, denial, anger, bargaining and acceptance. Fitchett in his 1981 paper to the Fourth Annual Conference of the National Hospice Organization, entitled, "Test the Validity of Kubler Ross' Stage Theory" suggested that this stage theory stereotyped death and dying counseling. I have been at times shocked to hear Social Workers trying to force a dying or bereaved person through those five stages (in that order) to acceptance. It has been suggested that there are tensions in confronting a personal death: resistance and acceptance. You will note that the earlier mentioned emotions all fall into the resistance category.

Resistance is a coping mechanism of coming to grips with their own death from cancer. Initially they are necessary to prevent the patient and the relatives from being overwhelmed and psychologically destroyed by something they are not prepared to accept. Resistance provides a buffer zone between a robust healthy life and impending death through cancer.

Any person, who would be a care provider for a dying person, must have previously dealt with their own journey through this buffer zone. There is no need to have had a terminal illness to pass through it. The need is for serious contemplation about your own death in an accident or through illness. Imagine yourself in one or other death or dying situation

My own such confrontation was in a dream which saw me in the operating theatre where I had an arrest and clinically died. My spirit left my body and rose to the ceiling and watched at they tried to resuscitate me and then pronouncing me dead. It was very real and I felt the experience and in a fashion I tasted death. What I experienced matched the stories of a number of near-death experiences that I have listened to. (I prefer not to use 'near-death experience' because it is a 'clinical death experience')

> *Resistance is a coping mechanism of coming to grips with their own death from cancer.*

Twelve months ago, I had a heart attack followed by Angioplasty and a quadruple bypass. At no time did my fearless, peaceful, trusting equilibrium leave me. Being comfortable with facing your own death should be a requirement for a pastoral care visitor to cancer or other dying patients.

The Care Offered

Being comfortable with your own death, means that with empathy, you are able to accept that the patient is dying or under threat. You are able to tolerate the sadness of the patient as he or she enumerates the persons or things they will be leaving behind. There is a tension between the inevitable and the desire to retain those tangible elements which have made up their life and made it meaningful. That tension expresses itself in many ways. In the period after the diagnosis, the good and the hurtful, the happy and the boring, the joyous and the calamitous, the easy and the hard times flash through the mind. Some of them are as clear as if they happened only a day or two ago. These recollections fill the patient with mixed emotions. All of these are going to be lost.

Perhaps some of the personalities will be waiting for them in the after life.

The carer has to quickly try to determine where those reminiscences had brought them as you arrived at the bedside. One of my points in the advocacy of full time chaplaincy to specific units of the hospital was that in three consecutive days the mood of the patient may vary each day because of the disease, the treatment, reaction to visitors or these memory recalls. By daily seeing the patient, different issues are able to be dealt with. So, the casual pastoral care visitor must quickly try to ascertain where the patient is at the time of that particular visit. Often, you cannot take up where you left off on your previous visit.

Remember the patient will be exhibiting the natural emotional responses to where they are at that particular moment. It is important for the carer to let the patient air their current feelings. It may be sadness over past events, regret over previous actions, and guilt over things they did or should have done. At other times it may be happiness recalling days of joy, blessing, lightheartedness, amusing episodes or the anticipation of realizing their faith's future reward.

The Carer's Role

The task of offering pastoral care to a cancer patient is serious and important, demanding an alertness which cannot afford to let concentration lapse. I have known patients to catch visitors out who have been inattentive in their listening by saying something is black to get a nod of agreement and then a few minutes later to say the opposite and get the same response. The pastoral visitor must keep the wits sharpened all the time. So the visitor must have good listening skills and have sufficient self-control so as not to interject and change the subject because it is uncomfortable to hear, deeply personal or other matters relating to the patient, his or her family, friends, or even church people. A non-shockable or non-judgmental assessment of the patient's story should always be shown.

A cancer patient often expects a pastoral visitor to know something about human life, its meaning and intent, its purpose and where it is headed. These are often topics which trouble the patient. If the patient raises these and like issues, there is a need to sensitively align them with the patient's current situation and if known and relevant to the patient's past history. In such situations, the carer must seek to extract the expression of the negative emotions and thinking which has generated the enquiry. Initially, this is more important than trying to introduce and arouse positive notions. The negative must be aired before any positive acceptance is possible. Carers must discard the maxim that their role is primarily to cheer the patient. A patient cannot be cheered while there are underlying, unresolved troubling issues.

To put it simply, the pastoral person's role is to clear the decks of the patient's life of any scum that might hinder a peaceful departure from this life. If the carer has not the skills to do this, then an appropriate referral should be made while there is time.

The Needed Qualities of the Carer

To meet the cancer patient's expectations, the carer needs to:
- show respect for the patient
- display appreciation of who the patient is
- listen with a discerning ear
- affirm the offer of understanding, concern, care and support
- encourage a realistic and positive hope.

To do this, the carer's ministry must be:
- flexible to the changing emotions and condition of the patient
- a supportive presence that is dependable
- able to respect the uniqueness of the patient, particularly as a cancer patient
- able to confront the patient concerning relationships, personal and spiritual matters, if necessary, and to be diplomatic and discrete in doing so
- treat each visit as a new situation without any set agenda
- allow the patient to raise any issue they desire to air.

The fruits of pastoral care may be negated by overtly, even zealously, trying to force or coerce the patients into certain actions of a religious or personal nature against their will. The carer must view ministry to the dying and in particular the cancer victim as a most sacred and responsible ministry of the church. It is a ministry which will never be truly successful unless the carer is daily renewed within him or herself by communion with God. The awareness of a personal closeness to the Divine enables the Holy Spirit to direct the visitor's footsteps at the appropriate time to the patient. In addition, the carer will become aware that the words which flow from the mouth are dictated by the Holy Spirit. Many have been the times when the words which poured from my lips sprang from nowhere else but by the dictation of God himself. Many pastoral workers have rushed in with talk on deeper spiritual issues only to be rebuffed because it was the wrong timing. The spirit not only gives the right words but it only gives them at the most appropriate time. Then and then only are the words able to be accepted by the patient because the patient has reached a suitable stage of spiritual awareness and receptivity

Thus, the pastoral visitor to a cancer patient must be spiritually prepared, abandoning self-confidence in self resources and allow the Holy Spirit to control the topics and trend of the encounter.

A Spiritual Ministry

The true pastoral person recognizes that God is no less working when his name is mentioned or not. The message of religion particularly as Jesus taught it, is love or in Islamic terms, compassion. God accompanies the spiritually attuned person to each bedside or home. The love or compassion of the carer which originates in God is conveyed to the patient whether God's name is mentioned or not. God is able to reveal himself through true pastoral care. When it is appropriate to mention God and the patient's relationship with God, there arises the opportunity for open spiritual communication. The patient's background may have built up resentment toward God and religion. The discerning carer depends upon God's spirit working in the patient to recognize that this love and compassion being shown is from God. This may be described as covert spiritual communication.

The physical, mental and religious background should determine whether God's love, mercy and forgiveness is explicitly a trend of the conversation or whether the more effective spiritual exercise is to allow the implicit Godly presence to be revealed through the pastoral visitor. In all pastoral visits to a cancer patient, it is God's spirit alone who ultimately opens the spiritual eyes of the patient to the presence, peace, comfort and love being expressed through the one providing the pastoral care.

For the cancer patient, bewildered and confused, a copy of the Serenity Prayer by Reinhold Neibuhr may be the most valuable contribution, you are able to make on a particular visit. It may raise issues that the cancer patient needs to deal with privately and perhaps later with a spiritual carer...For the carer, St. Francis of Assisi's Peace Prayer would be appropriate to use in preparing before each pastoral visit. Most religious book stores stock cards with these prayers on them.

Serenity Prayer

Grant me
The serenity to accept the things I cannot change,
The courage to change the things I can,
And the wisdom to know the difference.
Reinhold Niebuhr

Peace Prayer

Lord, make me an instrument of your peace.
Where there is hatred, let me sow love.
Where there is injury, pardon.
Where there is doubt, faith.
Where there is despair, hope.
Where there is darkness light.
Where there is sadness, joy.

Divine master, grant that I may not so much seek

To be consoled as to console;
To be understood, as to understand;
To be loved as to love;
For it is in giving that we receive,
It is in pardoning that we are pardoned,
It is in dying that we are born to eternal life.
St. Francis of Assisi.

CHAPTER 7

Digging

Into

Depression

As this book is basically a guide for pastoral visitors, I have been reluctant to deal with the question of despondency or depression. In this 21st century, in one form or another, depression is in all strata of society and age groups. Even pre-schoolers may be identifiably depressed. It is not a new phenomenon. However, it is more prevalent today.

A depressed person is constantly filled with suspicion, seeing only pessimistic outcomes. A depressed person is often recognized by having persistent low moods which are produced by stressful and harmony-destroying intrusions. A pre-school child expects, love, attention, affection, the necessities of life and sufficient personal quality time in a convivial atmosphere from its parents. A normal pre-school would accept reasonable chastisement for wrongdoing as a normal act of parental care. However, in this post-modern society, when both parents are working or are separated, the children see less and less of their parents. Babysitters or child care centers often have more to do with the child and are more able to listen to their problems. At home, the tired parent or parents often stressed from work as well as home responsibilities, are strained, and resort to shouting over trivial things with little opportunity to show and display affection. The child may become frightened, uncertain and even hide when hostile voices are raised. Instead of being happy and excited when the parent or parents come home, the child become agitated and reacts with attention-seeking dramatic outbursts or remains sullen and withdrawn in the hope of getting a hug and kiss. So from an early age a child may develop periods of low moods and negative assumptions about life.

A depressive illness may be recognized by withdrawn and negative moods and or fluctuating mood swings. It also affects a person's thinking and attitude to what is happening around them, as well as having physical effects on the body. True depression cannot be brushed aside as a temporary period of having the blues because of some isolated adverse event in the life of the person. Depression is much more serious and longer lasting. Unless treated, a depressive disorder can persist for years or ends tragically in suicide, drug abuse or alcoholism or other form of harmful thrill-seeking escape outlet.

> *A depressive illness may be recognized by withdrawn and negative moods and or fluctuating mood swings.*

The seriousness of depression is seen in figures produced by the U.S. National; Institute of Mental Health in its booklet entitled "Depression", issued in 2000. In any one year, 9.5% of Americans will suffer depression. The National Institute of Health in its fact sheet, dated May 03 2002, states that one fourth of women and one in eight men will suffer at least one onset of depression in their life time. It also estimates that three to five percent of all teenagers will experience clinical depression in any one year. Williams[10] cites (Paykel 1989) who states that four to five percent of Britons will suffer clinical depression at any one time. He takes the 1981 study of Amenson and Lewinsohn who suggest that ten percent will have

---

[10] Williams. J. Mark. G. *The Psychological Treatment of Depression* (Routledge:1992) p.4.

a depressive episode. Thus, we see that British and American evidence of depression is about the same.

Depression has intruded into the population in significant numbers.

Symptoms of Depression.

In visiting a home or a patient in hospital, it is necessary to be able to understand the symptoms of depression. Often, it is the pastoral visitor, (who knows the family and the person well), who is the first to recognize the symptoms. Depression is more than just the occasional feeling downcast and unhappy with the world as it is.

The various medical and professional counseling groups are almost unanimous in their list of the signs of depression. It may be noticed in a person who expresses feelings of or talk about being:
- Sad or empty
- Guilty, hopeless or pessimistic
- Worthless, useless or helpless
- Listless and having lost their former drive and initiative
- Unable to enjoy former pleasurable activities and things
- Unable to make decisions
- Unable to concentrate
- Irregular sleep patterns such as falling asleep, staying asleep, fitful sleeping, unable to sleep or difficulty in getting up.
- Troubled by aches and pains such as headaches, stomach and back pains, joint and muscle pains
- Irritable, angry, or continuously anxious

It is generally accepted, that when a person has five or more of these symptoms for most of the time over a two week period or more, then depression should be considered. It is confirmed when a person has bouts of the symptoms or fluctuating high or low mood swings.

Types of Depression

Like many physical or psychological illnesses, depression manifests itself in various forms. It is identified in three forms with various symptoms, periods of occurrence and severity. These three forms are Major Depression, Dysthymia, and Adjustment Disorder with Depressed mood.

A Major Depression is indicated when a combination of five or more of the above symptoms show themselves at anyone time, disenabling the sufferer to effectively study, work, sleep, eat, or derive pleasure from normally enjoyable activities. It may occur once only or several times during a person's life. At the time of occurrence, it is very disruptive for family and associates.

Dysthymia   is a less severe but chronic form of depression which is long term and not as dysfunctional or socially affecting as a major depression.

Adjustment Disorder with Depressive Moods occurs after a life shattering or changing event. It may be the result of a death, relationship breakdown, or other grief causing loss, including accidents, robbery, unemployment, financial problems, or failure of one sort or other etc. This form of depression is diagnosed when the ability to settle after the episode is prolonged and interferes with a person's ability to function normally. In some cases it may be called "unresolved grief".

These symptoms are not to be confused with the psychiatric condition Bipolar Disorder commonly referred to as *Manic Depressive. Manic Depression* involves bouts of major depression with periods of abnormally high moods and hyperactivity followed by   negative withdrawn despondency, irritability, anger or non-communication. These swings move from one extreme of the mood pendulum to the other. It is generally considered to be the result of a chemical imbalance in the brain and requires treatment from a psychiatrist. It must be recognized as being a psychiatric illness and should not be considered or dealt with as the other three depressions already mentioned.

Who Are Depression Sufferers?

There is no group that is immune from depression. We have already noted that in any one year, ten percent of the population is likely to suffer a bout or several fits of depression. When we consider that many of these may only have one attack of major depression in their entire lives, the total number who will experience depression will be several times the annual average. Hence it must be accepted that depression is a reasonably common condition requiring understanding care and treatment. Thus, it is important that pastoral visitors are aware of some of the facts about depression.

Gender Susceptibility As we have already seen women are more likely to be treated for depression than men. For many women, hormonal changes revolving around menstrual functions, natal and post-natal experiences can precipitate depressive episodes. Bilkon M.D. and Oren, D. A. in their article "Gender differences in Depression" in "Medscape Women's Health" 1997 - 2:3 emphasize that some forms of depression are common in new mothers. However, they claim that post-natal depression is not common but should have active intervention when it occurs. Post-natal depression has serious effects not only on the mother but also on the infant, which also impacts on the father and other members of the family.

Williams[11] comments on other research findings that suggest that young mothers with young children are more likely to become depressed because of the tension between paid or career employment and their role as an unpaid child carer.

We should not lose sight of the fact that men are able to mask their depression more easily than women and that they are sometimes reluctant to admit and seek professional help for their depression. Men are able to escape from the home and its tensions to the public bar or club to drink with their mates. Under the influence of the alcohol, the depression is drowned until the effects wears off. The mother has few opportunities for such a relief from the pressure of home and family.

Let us, now, look at Depression in children, adolescents and adults.

---

[11] Williams 1992 p.6.

Depression in Children

Any child from toddler to adolescence shows sadness from time to time. Often it is in response to some trauma or negative experience. Normal sadness is of short duration. Depressive sadness in children often lasts much longer. At times, it is in conjunction with unusual irritability both, inside and outside the home, disagreement with play mates, changes in behavioral patterns and learning problems at school. The possibility of one or other forms of depression should be considered when the symptoms remain unchanged or deteriorate over any period longer than two weeks.

Care must be taken not to confuse this with attention-deficit disorder and hyperactivity (ADHD) which requires the help of psychiatry and medication. Often, children are wrongfully diagnosed with ADHD when it is bipolar-disorder or manic-depression. A pastoral visitor can easily get out of their depth and make unjustified assumptions which may offend the parents of the child. Therefore, the pastoral carer should not appear to be the expert. The pastoral visitor is not expected to be a diagnostician. He or she should be sufficiently alert to a problem and suggest the pursuit of appropriate professional consultation. Even then, care must be exercised where it is perceived that the parents are denying that there is anything out of the ordinary with their child.

Depression in a child should be taken seriously as it affects the child's social, physical and educational development. This includes self-esteem and self-confidence both essential for a happy and successful future life.

A depressed child under six years may have a perpetually sad face and only with great difficulty can it be stimulated to extract a grudging smile. They may have difficulty in having fun and show reluctance to join others of similar age who are enjoying themselves. To see themselves as hopeless and useless at that age becomes an ingrained outlook on life which unless professionally treated will end in disaster or self-destruction. The loss of self-esteem generated by this dysthymia is evidence of the child's feelings of personal ugliness, unloveableness, stupidity, and inability to do normal things for their age. This leads to developmental retardation and a reluctance to try to achieve in any area of life.

A child suffering from depression may be susceptible to persistent fits of crying for no apparent or little reason for doing so. A depressed child may have a preoccupation with death and even talk of suicide. Many parents take scant regard to such talk. The child's threat of suicide may be an attention-seeking plot or it may be a dare. If the dare is ignored or brushed aside, it may be acted on with dire consequences. An attention-seeking plot such as this has some underlying cause which must be traced as early as possible to avoid a tragedy.

A child suffering from bipolar disorder or manic depression presents with the following symptoms which should be taken seriously:
- Extreme hyperactivity, effervescent non-stop activity from early morning until bed-time
- This contrast with periods of moroseness and self deprecations
- Sudden and rapid mood swings between the above two
- Frequent and prolonged explosive temper tantrums or rages.
- Over confidence in self and abilities.

An unwillingness to accept that a child may have bipolar disorder often results in a diagnosis of attention-deficit disorder with hyperactivity (ADHD), or obsessive –compulsive disorder.

Causes of Childhood Depression
- There may be a family history of depression
- Having different interests from other children
- Being subject to school bullying for being smart or slow with school work, not being a robust sporting type, have some prominent physical feature such as big nose, ears etc.
- A significant death in the family such as grandparent, parent, sibling or playmate or kindly neighbor
- Divorce of parents can be a major trigger of insecurity, unrealistic self-blame for the separation, or longing for reconciliation may turn normal sadness into depression

- Clinical depression may relate to the functioning of the neuro-transmitters in the brain that regulate mood and endorphins that affect the production of positive moods
- Irrational guilt over the presumed effects of something they said or did
- Insufficient love, protection and recognition within the family
- Sexual, physical or verbal abuse in the home

Action to Be Taken

If the previously noted symptoms apply to the child then the parents should:

- Be keenly observant of the child's behavior
- Detail in writing behavioral changes, duration of those changes, their frequency and how seriously they seem
- Contact a mental health professional for evaluation and diagnosis
- Research reliable sources for information concerning childhood mental health to understand the child
- Be persistent with questions, about the diagnosis and treatment, to the professional

Pastoral Intervention.

A pastoral carer can do little in the area of professional treatment or counseling of the child. This often requires long term therapy and should be the prerogative of a professional. The pastoral visitor should have some idea of the signs and symptoms of depression as they have been itemized. Where a major depression or dysthymia are suspected, it must be recognized and accepted by the visitor and parents that the child possibly needs psychotherapy and /or medication. Therapy enables the child to deal with the problematic issues.

It must be remembered that an untreated depressed child will have long term effect upon the family and life long repercussions for the child. The seriousness of childhood depression should not be underestimated. If possible, the pastoral responsibility is to diplomatically ensure that the parents are aware of this. If the parents are financially stretched, then, arrangements should be made for private or church support toward the expenses.

The carer must be unfailing in the support of the parents during this time, showing interest, care and concern for the child. This may be by cooperating with the parents and the church to see that the child is involved in interests outside the home. This will enable the child to fraternize with other children and divert the mind off themselves to other interesting activities.

The pastoral visitor is able to offer helpful advice to the parents to:
- Show love to the child
- Avoid shouting at the child by not over reacting to misbehavior
- Listen to what the child is saying or trying to say
- If the parental relations with the child are strained, encourage the child to talk with a relative, sibling, close family friend or suitable other confidant.
- Draw out the child's feelings both happy and unhappy without showing negative reactions. It is best just to let the child talk.
- Encourage the parents to seek help of a child psychologist or psychiatrist preferably a pediatric psychiatrist.
- The parents might be advised to see a family counselor to consider their role in the depression and how they can help the situation.
- Reassure the parents that depression is curable.

Childhood depression is a condition. A person with a pastoral heart who does not try to assume the role of therapist is able to provide real assistance to the child and family by being caring, supportive and encouraging, even when, at times, the support may not be welcome. The carer's sincerity and ability to get alongside the family at their level usually wins out.

Depression in a Teenager

In most western countries, people are critical of the present day teenagers and young people. They are often seen moving in small groups or larger gangs and are responsible for unsightly graffiti, wanton acts of vandalism and the destruction of personal, public and private property. These are in the minority yet get the lion share of teenage media publicity. By comparison, most teenagers are contented, conscientious, well-balanced and productive.

Somewhat disturbing statistics have been produced[12] suggesting that by the age of 21 years, ten to twenty percent have had a major depressive episode. They state that 35% of younger women will have shown evidence of major depression. The "W.H.O. Health Policy for Children and Adolescence" shows that in the U.S. in 1997-98 of those age fifteen years, 49% of females and 34% of males reported weekly depressive episodes.[13] The policy report surveys 28 countries and shows the U.S. with the highest incidence. There may be cultural, educational and other factors which contribute to the variation in figures between the countries.

We do not have to look far for the reasons as to why teenagers are susceptible to depression.

The beginning of the teen years marks the onset of puberty and hormonal changes. At this age the nature of education takes a step or two higher as more responsibility is expected from them as they move from primary to secondary education. Teenage body changes and development as well as educational expectations are adding new and different responsibilities which impose previously unencountered pressure on them.

---

[12] Lewinsohn P.M., Clarke G.N. (1999) Psychosocial treatments for adolescent depression. Clin Psychol Rev 19(3):329-324
[13] WHO Policy Series: Health policy for children and adolescents, International Report 1:39-45. Copenhagen Denmark: WHO) 2000

Puberty brings altered perceptions of the opposite sex. Previously they were a boy or girl by the accident of conceptual birth and generally boys and girls saw things differently and had different interests. As the body changes, an awareness of anatomical differences and functions are now being realized. They see the opposite sex through different eyes. Knowledge and understanding of sexual function arouses curiosity and so thoughts of experimentation arise-often against parental mores. Thus more pressure is applied.

However, in the more permissive societies like the U.S., European and Australian cultures, many of the former moral standards and expectations have been relaxed in some areas. This makes it easier for teenagers to conform to peer pressure and breakaway from adult social conventions of fifty years ago. The rules and convention of previous generations are able to be broken and flouted. Sensitivity to acceptance and rejection is heightened in this period.

Success or failure can lead to the type of peers with whom a teenager associates. The natural gregarious instincts to belong and conform to herd norms dominate this period. This conformity rule adds further pressure. Being less that successful means that they have to link up with like underachievers, hence the development of the group or gang mentality to show strength and power.

These underachievers take up anti-social stances which develop further their low-self esteem and sense of inferiority rather than giving a positive boost to their ego. They tend to be involved in outrageous attention seeking behavior to raise their image as a person who can do things. Their achievements are destructive. When alone in their more reflective moments they are prime candidates for depression. The gang strikes give them a weird sense of achievement or their solo hits are their way

in the more permissive societies like the U.S., European and Australian cultures, many of the former moral standards and expectations have been relaxed in some areas.

of being further bogged down in a sense of futility about their lives. Often, the courage to perform these eye-catching public exploits is gained from ingestion of alcohol or drugs.

In many households, the teenager desires to extend the boundaries that child and family upbringing have imposed. Being neither man nor boy, woman nor girl, they are unable to understand why parental wisdom and discipline should be acknowledged and accepted. Thus, many teenagers begin to rebel against family, restrictions, regulations and directions. This rebellious spirit they take into their school and against all others who are in a position of authority

There are other factors which can lead to teenage depression. One of the most significant is the interplay of family relations. If one or other parent is depressed it is possible for the teenager to develop it. In families where one or both parents are authoritarian, strict disciplinarians or perfectionists, the children feel that they are not able to meet up with their parents' high standards. Their failure to please their parents often means that they give up trying.   They see their sense of failure at home as prophetic of how they will fare in the future. Where a parent or parents are nonchalantly slovenly in the home, the teenager is likely to feel ashamed to invite their friends to their home because of the state of the house. Embarrassed at not being able to reciprocate hospitality, they feel they are not good enough to be a friend of their peers, and so, withdraw. The machinery for the development of the characteristics of depression were set in motion in the home as a pre-teen and reached crescendo by mid-teens.

A home in which marital harmony and affection is or was non-existent, or the parents separated and divorced, the teenager can build up resentment toward one or both parents. The lies, the innuendos, breach of trust, insecurity and denial of love and true affection by both parents may leave the teenager feeling left out on a limb and uncertain as to what will happen next.   Often, this broken trust in adults is difficult to restore; so, the lonely, resentful, angry young person falls a prey to depression. The teenager's resilience to it has been eroded.

Teenage depression is often dysthymic that is chronic and long lasting with frequent relapses.

Symptoms of Teenage Depression

A depressed teenager shows any combination of the previously identified general symptoms of depression. However, there are a number of significantly other important indicators. These additional traits include:
- Noticeable difficulty in dealing with routine responsibility
- Alcohol and substance abuse
- Poor concentration
- Degenerating performances in school or other activities
- Truancy from school
- Running away from home
- Deliberately ignoring time commitments at home or school
- Threat of suicide or death
- Obsession with poor body and face image.
- Liability to withdraw into themselves – the loner
- Females prone to anorexia and bulimia.

Action to Be Taken

Parents should take the same action as for a depressed child. Parents and friends must realize that trying to cheer them up will not help the suicide or depressed mood to go away. The parents need to talk with the parents of other teenage children. This will help them to understand the ethos of the teenagers and therefore be better equipped to communicate and help their own adolescent. There are family network organizations in the community facilitated by professional youth specialists. These should be joined to gain insights for supporting their young person. In addition, networking will provide the parents with opportunities to compare their own current personal problems as well as dealing with their grief over their teenager's unhealthy state.

Pastoral Perception

Similar guidelines apply for pastoral engagement with a low-spirited teenager and the family as to a child. However, the teenager is a little different, in that the teenager may have a more developed emotional and intellectual background.

The pastoral person should always be accepting of the young person. It is critical that the carer's kindness, love, and guarantee of continuing support are recognized. A teenager smothered by low self-esteem, lack of self confidence, humiliated by peer group taunts, feeling isolated and full of despair needs that assurance particularly from the carer with the home encouraged to do the same. Their sense of shame, unlovableness and perhaps guilt make it difficult for them to express themselves in words. Spend time with them, at first, often mostly in acceptable silence. When words are offered that are positive and assuring, a thaw starts to melt the frigidity and words start to trickle out from the one depressed. Further, careful, non-judgmental, listening will increase the flow.

Only after several serious attempts at revealing times of such talking should any recommendation be made for professional help. To suggest such help too soon may strengthen their depressive state. If possible, some form of trust should be gained first. This principle should be curtailed if there is repeated talk of death or suicide. Even if the carer is pressed to tell no one of the suicide threat, the parents and a professional should be alerted. Such a promise may mean the saving of a life or many lives. If the perpetrators of the Columbine High and Red Lake School massacres had been listened to, these tragedies may have been avoided. Those dealing with depressed young people must keep in mind that the rate of teenage suicide has increased in the last few decades. It is a major concern.

Where a youth clings to the belief that depression shows a weakness or warped personality and character, this fallacy should be countered by pointing out the positives the young person   presently has and the potentials for a bright future. The myth of no hope for a depressed person should be squashed by repeatedly affirming that, with help, depression is curable and a normal productive life should be envisioned.

A Depressed Adult

In adulthood the pressures of living in society vary from those experienced in childhood and adolescence. In those pre-adult years, a person is mostly living in an inter-dependent family relationship where most of the burden and responsibility for daily needs fall upon the parents. The norm is that, in adulthood, the provisions for life are cast upon the now independent adult. Often, there may be added the load of caring for spouse, children and aging parents.

Fifty years ago, behavioral psychiatrists showed a strong inclination to see depression as biological in which the typical characteristics of depression were the behavioral effects of chemical imbalance which was treatable with anti-depressive drugs. Those with bipolar or manic depression fall into this category.

The more common forms of depression are *endogenous and reactive depressions.* The former is due to a chemical imbalance and is able to be controlled by medication.

The latter form of depression is the reactive response to external stressful experiences and circumstances. These depressions arise as the result of the internalized reaction to external stresses.

Most of the depressed people that may be encountered in pastoral visitation would be this non-biological or reactive type. It must be remembered that they also may need some medication along with psychotherapy; hence the importance of seeking a professional referral.
There is merit in being able to understand this type of reactive depression as being the result of some external, disturbing intrusion into the life of the depressed. Certainly a traumatic loss through death or other means as already mentioned my precipitate a depressive condition. Part of the human psyche expects what is known as social reinforcement to function normally in society. This is part of the gregarious or herd instinct within us. We need a continuing sense of approval and encouragement from society if we are to maintain a good stimulus for living.

In childhood and teens, doting parents, grandparents, family, teachers, and friends often provided positive and encouraging complimentary strokes on the younger person. This provides the incentive to please adults, achieve good grades in school or in the fields of arts or sport. Where such positive reinforcement is not forthcoming a child is likely to become moody and even depressed. In adults this need for positive reinforcement is perhaps more essential. Self-achievement in business or any other enterprise thrives on appreciation and acclaim. When a person such as a spouse is taken for granted and their promotion, tidy house, gourmet cuisine, colorful garden etc are not recognized and applauded the seeds for depression as well as divorce are sown. In cases where a person's behavior or efforts are unworthy of recognition or appreciation then such recognition is not possible. The person has no reason to feel pleased with themselves or their efforts. They remain unrecognized and again the soil is being readied for depression. Humans have a need for social reinforcement and encouragement to recognize, pursue and further the gifts that they already possess.

Those whose self esteem is not strong, possibly because of their pre-adult years, have minimal social reinforcement. Many try hard to please and be accepted by the social group. Not to be accepted or not to be part of the inner circle, to them, is a form of punishment such as they felt in childhood. This desire to please creates a sense of anxiety as they make special efforts. Anxiety is considered a component of depression, even mild depression. When those efforts go unacknowledged, they fire up more intense feelings of uselessness, further anxiety, anger with society and other traits of depression. The desire to persist to please and belong to society is abandoned as depression continues to take over their lives and outlook on life. Less self-assured and frustrated parents of rebellious teenagers are candidates for such development.

An adult with fewer achievements than those of their group and married to a person with either higher or lower social status or who has a deficit in social skills is likely to feel the odd person and unable to participate in the conversations of the group. Another person may be able to express themselves in conversation but have the ability to put their foot in their mouth, causing repeated upsets. They may have the self-confidence but may alienate others by saying or doing the wrong thing at the wrong time. Such repeated experiences push them to the outer circle. Repeated rebuttal or rejections causes them to withdraw into themselves and become depressed. These people have failed to learn from their experiences to control their speech and action.

Consequently, the depressed person becomes passive toward society. Their lack of ability to control their behavior or improve their social skills or knowledge leaves them with a sense of futility toward life and of their ability to make any changes to their situation. Persons meeting with reactively depressed people must remember that it is a learned condition from experience. Anything learned can be unlearned by right tuition and guidance.

This unlearning tuition should be given by professional practitioners who will probably use cognitive therapy. An inexperienced person may produce another failure and a greater and more desperate depressed condition. Cognitive therapy enables the patient to recognize the origins and the reasons why their behavior has put them into their depressed state. With such recognition they are able to readjust their thinking and restructure their way of behaving towards others. Where low self-esteem has been the contributing factor, the person will recognize the underutilized talents and develop others.

Where depression is caused by loss, rejection, childhood abuse, unacknowledged worthy efforts, relationship breakdown, guilt, embarrassment, shame or other causes, all these are able to be scrutinized in cognitive therapy   which is beyond the normal pastoral person's capability or role.

It will be noted that I have not dealt with depression in the elderly as this is a subject in itself. It is in part covered in my "Pastoral Care to the Aged" Morehouse 2005.

Pastoral Perception

As we have so frequently stated, a professional referral is essential for depressed persons. It may be necessary to accompany the person to the professional for the first few visits until the patient gains sufficient self-confidence to go alone. Such accompaniment should not be offered if a sympathetic, responsible family member is able to go with them. The family should be involved in the restoration and rehabilitation.

A pastoral person, perhaps, with the help of a church group to whom the patient may be introduced or the pastoral carer alone may be able to:

- encourage the patient to do some small tasks they have not been doing – assisting until they can do it by themselves
- gradually increase the difficulty of the tasks
- take them out of their environment on outings, picnics, movies, sporting fixtures, concerts or other activities that might take their interest
- go for walks or do other light exercise with them
- pay compliments and give praise for progress or achievement – social; reinforcement
- continually reassure them of a cure remembering that a diagnosis of bipolar or manic depressive is permanent and medication must continue.
- continually enquire about and encourage them to persist with the doctor's instructions concerning medication and alcohol products.
- any talk of suicide should be reported to the practitioner
- constantly reassure the patient of your continuing support

Depression is a serious condition which an active pastoral person will undoubtedly encounter. Where rapport and trust has been developed with the depressed patient being visited, the relationship must be maintained. Failure to do so may be seen as a further rejection.

Be cautious in case you go beyond your ability to be of use. Willingness to seek assistance from a more skilled practitioner should be maintained.

Any ministry to a depressed person should always be backed by the seeking of an awareness of the Divine Spirit's guidance and presence.

The following are extracts of a statement by a person, I know, who suffered temporary depression. She was a very outgoing person and had experienced one of those external intrusions which shattered her.

"I was given the name of a specialist psychiatrist... a sweet person from the church would run me to his rooms and wait for me.... A friend from the church who had been through a similar experience was of great help...they offered me a bed in their home at any time or just to call in and I did that many times.... Even though I felt pain because of the contrast which had happened so suddenly in my life, I couldn't appreciate at the time the cards, the phone calls, and love that came in bunches of flowers which made me cry, I really underneath loved everyone and would go over the words of the cards or letters, knowing that people loved me, as much as when I was well and able to help others....

Don't tell about how you know what the other person is going through because your mother has had five nervous breakdowns! That will only make the person feel and think the worst that it is going to keep happening! No, be very careful to be positive. The words that helped me were those like 'this is only temporary, it will pass, you will get better.' Positive bible verses such as those about God being stronger and especially about God being a healer are wonderful.....

Everyone has different reasons for their illness, but it is just as real an illness when it happens, and I think the help the church people can give those who have reached this stage of stress is needed right now. If the church doesn't bring Christ's comfort and hope to those in need, then other institutions can only dab the surface and help in a human and humane way..... We are body, mind and spirit and when one of these is affected all are affected, so we need to look after them.....and I am praising Him for my good health restored.

One of the several traumatic incursions into the life of the writer at the time was the diagnosis of a beloved grandchild with brain tumor and the subsequent surgery and chemotherapy."

CHAPTER 8

The Spirit
Of
Forgiveness

A Jewish parable on forgiveness tells of a king who had a vehement disagreement with his son. The confrontation was so bitter that the king banished his son from the kingdom. For years, the son roamed from country to country unhappy, miserable and bitter.

As the years passed, the king began to have remorse over the exiling of his son. Emissaries were sent to all the countries around to seek him out, offering him forgiveness and an invitation to return to the royal household.

After much searching, the son was located and the invitation extended to accept the forgiveness and to return to his home. The son's bitterness was so great that he would not return nor would he accept his father's forgiveness, responding with very unpleasant and abusive language. The heartbroken king sent a compromise that they meet half way to talk things over and come to some reconciliation. The resentful heart of the son again refused the offer of conciliation.

The story does not tell us what the son did to deserve being exiled. The hurting son, no doubt, felt his punishment was totally unjustified. His father thought otherwise and issued the son-interpreted loveless, unforgiving order of exile.

Let us link this with two other parables also told by a Jew. Jesus spoke of a son who demanded his inheritance and exiled himself from home until he had reaped in full the fruit of his hurtful, selfish and unloving spirit toward his father. In the depths of his own self-created misery he admitted the wrong done against his father. So with deep remorse, he set out to seek his father's forgiveness. The compassionate father was longing and waiting for his son to return and instantly forgave him. The stay-at-home, self righteous, obedient elder brother resented his reinstatement into the household. Even with his father's entreaties and expressions of love, this brother remained outside the house, a resentful, bitter, unforgiving person.

The third parable, also told by Jesus, tells of a court official who borrowed an extraordinary large amount of money from the king. Several years later, unable to repay his debt, the king granted him a full release from the debt - a most generous, unexpected and compassionate act.

This same court official then went out and put into a debtor's prison a fellow king's employee for his inability to repay a paltry debt. The king upon hearing this was so abhorred and enraged that he rescinded his generous offer to the ungrateful officer   and inflicted the full weight of the law for debt defaulters upon him

Identifying the Characters

Let us identify the characters in the three stories.

Parable 1.
- **1.** The king who exiled his son for unknown offences and later was willing to forgive the son.
- **2.** The exiled aggrieved resentful son whose hurt festered so much he refused the forgiveness offered.

Parable 2.

- **3.** A generous father who unnecessarily blessed his younger son and then waited for his return to forgive him.
- **4.** The selfish younger son who took what he could from the father and lived riotously. He returned a repentant son to seek his father's forgiveness.
- **5.** A self-righteous, stay a home, elder son who was bitterly jealous of his father's forgiving spirit could not forgive his brother.

Parable 3.
- **6.** The king who forgave an exorbitant debt of an employee,
- **7.** The forgiven official who refused to forgive a colleague a minor debt.
- **8.** A small debtor fellow employee who was sent to a debtors' prison by the unforgiving, forgiven king's official.

Characters 1, 3 and 6 are authoritarian figures that show a generosity of spirit and forgiveness to unworthy underlings.

Characters 2, 4 and 7 have been forgiven or offered forgiveness by their superior

Character 5 is unwittingly involved with the other two characters and according to the stories along with character 2 remained unforgiving and character 8 who was unforgiven.

As a pastoral visitor moves among people he or she will most probably meet all eight types who need forgiveness, need to exercise forgiveness, or remain unforgiven though not being offered forgiveness. Wherever humans meet, interact and communicate, their imperfect human nature will manifest, some will offend or otherwise hurt others, physically, emotionally materially or even spiritually. That harm may be intentionally or unintentionally inflicted.

Intentional harm may be inflicted through jealousy, ambition, malice, retaliation or plain selfishness. Words or actions may unintentionally cause sadness and sorrow, physical or emotionally, to another person. Such may be due to carelessness, ignorance, thoughtlessness, insensitivity, negligence or the prevailing circumstances often created by others.

Character 1 – The King Who Relented

In the first parable there are two characters and it may be divided into two episodes. In the first the king appears hard and unforgiving who exiles his son.

The king might be classed as a strong ruler. He was adamant that things be done decently and in order. He was a strict "letter of the law" administrator. He would not tolerate any breach of the moral and ethical code of his authority. Some might say he was an excessively severe custodian of his country's laws. He commanded and demanded respect due to his position. It was for this reason the country was efficiently and happily run.

> *Words or actions may unintentionally cause sadness and sorrow, physical or emotionally, to another person.*

For some reason his own son violated his strict code of conduct and behavior. They had a heated confrontation over it. It reached boiling point with neither king nor son relenting or compromising in any manner. The anger was so obvious and hostile that it became malevolent. The longer it raged, the more defiant the son became until the king had no alternative action to take. The son's pride would not allow him to seek forgiveness or say sorry for his breach of established convention.

The king was justified in his judgment that his son was worthy of being disinherited and exiled. The harsh sentence fits in with the contemporary saying, "if you do the crime, you do the time." The father was the one who was responsible to see the rules and laws of the land were maintained. Therefore, his son's actions demanded the full punishment of the law. It was a just and fair decision.

After some considerable time, the king was hurting within over the absence of the son. He was loaded with guilt over banishing his son from his presence. Here was a father realizing, in his aging years, the loss of the companionship and support of his own son in ruling the kingdom. He could bear it no longer, so, he set plans in motion to pardon or forgive his son. No doubt, he was hoping that the son had learned his lesson, had matured and would return to take his rightful place as a royal prince.

The notable thing about this king is that, although he was stringent in the application of the law, he was not without feeling and mercy. His decision, to offer clemency to his unruly, disrespectful son, was such a magnanimous act it would have drawn some unexpressed criticism from his senior advisors. They would have seen it as an unjustified back down against the king's own principles.

Such is the magnanimity of true forgiveness. It is offered when, seemingly, it is completely undeserved. The greatest expression of such high-minded benevolence is seen in God's willingness to recall men and women into his embrace by His forgiveness of their disobedience to His, God's, laws.

Such an offer was a triumph for the king. His authoritarian, hard heart had melted. It was now more loving, softer, conciliating and forgiving. The instant he made the decision to forgive, it was like the shedding of a huge burden. He was doing the right thing and moving in the right direction of peace and the restoration of his own inner harmony, irrespective of what his son did.

Character 3 - The Generous Father

The father in the second parable shows trust in his younger son. The son is now an adult and makes a request which in one respect is against the cultural norm. He asks his father for his share of the inheritance before his father's death. Instead of taking offence, the father grants the unusual plea. The son, by rights, should stay and work the father's estate with his brother, thereby meriting his share as an inheritance. Instead the father halves the assets selling what is necessary to give to the younger son. The father sees this as an opportunity for the son to prove that he is worthy of the chance to succeed in life on his own. The father puts confidence in his son.

After many years, the father's faith in the son is still as strong and he is constantly waiting for sign of the son's return home, even if only for a visit. He yearns to see his long lost beloved son. Then the selfish son returns and receives an undeserved hero's welcome home. Those wasted years of this now unpretentious failure as a person of integrity are all forgotten. Such is the generosity of this forgiving father.

As Jesus indicated, this father is comparable with the all loving, forgiving God. This God sets the example for all to follow. There is not a sinful act that God is unable to forgive, if that forgiveness is sought in the right spirit. God desires that we all have and maintain a forgiving spirit, however hard it must be to do so. We must remember that God forgives but does not condone the sin that is being forgiven.

Character 6. – The Debt Forgiving King

The king in the third parable is also a setter and administrator of rules and regulations. This king is also perceptive, merciful and generous. This generous kindliness is seen in his willingness, first of all, to trust his court officer by loaning a fortune in order to establish himself in life as an honorable and successful citizen. This officer proves untrustworthy, wasting his opportunity and finishing up bankrupt. The sympathetic king reviews the situation, assessing that the servant has lost everything and is facing extreme hardship, so, he forgives him of his debt. He even retains him on his staff and thereby giving him another chance. It was an unbelievable act of generosity which permitted him to retain his station within the kingdom without humiliation or disgrace. We also know that the officer again proved untrustworthy by refusing to forgive another of a small debt. So the kindly disposed king had to rescind the clemency on the ungrateful servant putting him in gaol until he could repay the huge debt.

The Three Forgiving Leaders.

In looking at these three men of authority, we see three types of forgiveness. The first offers forgiveness which is not accepted yet he leaves the offer on the table without any sign of grievance. This forgiving king shows a degree of patience and does not give up that his son may come to his senses and accept the offered forgiveness and return home.

The second offer of forgiveness is by a wealthy land owner to a reformed wasteful son. The father realized that the son made a courageous and risky decision to return home. What if the father had been unwilling to even accept him as a son? He took a risk but he also knew the nature of his father. He had seen his father in action with others who had offended the father when they sought reconciliation. He was a father of stable character who was unchanging in his dealings with men of all stations in life.

The third act of forgiveness was an incredible act of generosity to forgive such an enormous debt when it was so unnecessary to do so. The debt was forgiven in its entirety. Such generosity was unheard of in court or business circles. There wasn't even any need for negotiation or compromise. The expectation was that the officer would pattern his life and action upon that of the king. The king anticipated his forgiveness would beget forgiveness

These are parables but each show different ways by which God deals with humans. Remember! God put a tremendous amount of trust in us when we were made like him and able to make our own decisions. Each of the rulers offered forgiveness under very different circumstances. They also exemplify ways in which we are able to be free with our offers of forgiveness to those who have wronged or offended us.
Let us now look at the second set of characters in each parable.

Character No.2. The Exiled Son

We are not told of the reason for the father's hasty, harsh penalty. It must have been a very serious crime against his father and the kingdom. We do not know whether he was heir to the throne or a younger son who was plotting a coup because he realized his brother or brothers were in succession before him. It could only have been something very outrageous and criminal for a father to exile his son.

In exile, the son ponders over his lost opportunity. He squirms in the mire of his "poor me" syndrome. The son must have been missing the comforts of palace life and the privileged life of a prince. Increasingly, he became more and more bitter against his father. Not a day passed without being starkly reminded of the severity of his father's punishment of him, which he considered harsh and unjustified. As the months passed into years his resentment grew into a deeper and more resistant hatred.

The father's heart softened so he sent word offering forgiveness, restoration and reconciliation. The stubborn heart of the son remained unmoved except to consider that by refusing his father's approach, his father would be full of remorse to the end of his days. He saw his refusal as an act of revenge and somewhat gloated over the thought. Those years of brooding and contempt for his father could only be satisfied by him making his father suffer. This way it would be endless. In fact, the son gained a very macabre sense of justification

His father's second attempt at forgiveness and reunion suggested a meeting at a place half-way, for a face to face talk over the situation. This also met with a similar rebuttal. His anger against his father never went off the boil. His whole outlook on life became negative, warped and soul destroying. With bitterness and resentment fixed in his mind, it remained closed and became increasingly impossible for him to think objectively about it. The incessant reflecting on it turned him into a self-considered saint persecuted by an incarnate devil. He might be considered as looking continually into the mirror to adjust his saintly halo of innocence of any wrongdoing against his father. When his father's offer of forgiveness reached him he had the facts so distorted and twisted that the thought of acceptance was anathema.

This exiled son ended his days an unhappy, bitter man not experiencing the peace and luxury of his father's house that awaited him if he had accepted his father's overtures of forgiveness.

Character 4. The Selfish Son

Life was so good while he was lavishing his inheritance on wine, women and song and perhaps much gambling. He had money so there was no need to work. His new found friends were able to manipulate and cajole him into spreading his fortune around. In time, the good life had to come to an end. His money supply dried up and so did his partying friends. As his debts mounted so he had to seek employment to try and make repayments. In a poor country, where sons followed in their father's occupation jobs were scarce. Only the most menial employment that sons would not do was available to outsiders. Hence the repulsive, humiliating, degrading task of feeding pigs was the only employment available. His meager income was swallowed up by his debts so he was constantly hungry.

In his despair, he reflected on his life and what it would be like in his father's house. Even the father's servants were better off than he was. Unlike the exiled son, the selfish son viewed the situation from a larger canvas. He considered the reasons for his present predicament and that it was not his father's fault. He understood the cause of the wretchedness of his condition. It was his fault and he accepted responsibility for it. He acknowledged his own selfish stupidity. He considered what he should do about it.

He set off to return to his father, to confess his sinfulness, seek his father's forgiveness and request to work as a servant. He had no pretensions as to who he was. All pride had been beaten out of him. He considered himself unworthy of sonship and would fall on the mercy of his father to forgive him and employ him.

This selfish, now remorseful son did not count on his father's ability to continue to love him, nor the extent to which his father's mercy would stretch. When his father saw his wayward son's genuine humility and contriteness he restored him back to full sonship. The father discounted the calamitous nature of the son's sojourn and life in the far off country in showing the completeness of his forgiving act.

Character 7.

The Ungrateful Servant.

The exiled servant remained living in the alien land because of his self-righteous and unrelenting pride. The king's official who had his huge debt forgiven and wiped clean, had nothing to be aggrieved or angry about. He had every right to feel grateful and relieved at the lifting of this burden of debt. The fact that he had failed to capitalize on the king's generosity was no reason to let his frustration control his thinking. His gratitude was swamped by his wounded, puffed up pride which he felt could be overcome by a show of arrogant authority. His self-conceit became exaggerated by his reasoning that he must be indispensable to the king. This arrogance knew no bounds, so he lauded it over other members of the king's court.

There was a fellow servant who borrowed a paltry sum from him. This servant could not repay it fully by the due date so the forgiven servant had him sent to prison. Presumably, the onus to pay would have fallen on his relatives.

On hearing what his court officer, had done to a fellow officer the king was filled with wrath and was furious. The king immediately withdrew his forgiveness and imposed the same conditions of law upon the ungrateful servant as the ungrateful servant had applied to his fellow worker. Because of the enormity of the loan owing to the king, the ungrateful servant had the rest of his life to languish in jail contemplating the folly of ingratitude and false sense of egoistical pride.

3 Recipients of Offered Forgiveness

These three people, who had forgiveness offered them, are typical people we encounter in everyday life. Undoubtedly pastoral visitors will meet these three types when they move amongst people in the community. They each responded to the offer in different ways.

The exiled son was so bitter against his father that when the offer of forgiveness and reconciliation were offered he spurned it. He allowed the offer to further fuel his enmity toward his father who stretched out his hand in appeasement. He was presented with an opportunity to return to a privileged position which he was missing and desired above all else. It was a situation which would have restored him privilege, status, peace, friendship and other opportunities, otherwise unattainable. It was stubborn pride, ingrained bitterness and deep seated egotistical self-righteousness that would not allow him to accept his father's offer. He rejected forgiveness. He had built around himself a double defense against any armistice offer by his father. Unlike his father, he remained unforgiving, nursing a warped and bitter personality.

It was a twisted uncompromising reaction which was like a terminal illness of the spirit which he bore to the end of his days. He preferred to wallow in self-inflicted punishment and spirit of malingering hatred rather than lose face by returning back home to his father's love. Such people remain, bearing an unsociable morose, negative attitude to all of life and toward all people.

The selfish son was the reverse. Also in afar country, away from home and bereft of former home comforts, he considered the true reasons for his misery. His was an honest appraisal of his situation and why he was in it. He accepted responsibility for where he was. He recognized that he alone could get himself out of the mess. Anything would be better than feeding pigs and feeling like one. He decided to seek forgiveness and it was more than forgiveness he received.

The ungrateful servant was a user and would-be exploiter of people. He traded on the generous nature of the king for whom he worked. The king's willingness to help and trust his employees was expected to be rewarded with loyalty and similar generosity of spirit. The ungrateful servant was avaricious and self centered and cared little for the condition or needs of others. His attitude killed any opportunity for compassion or forgiveness to be exercised toward others.

Character 5 - The Stay-at-Home Son

The third person in the second parable is the elder son who loyally stayed at home working on his father's property which would be his inheritance. So, he virtually, was working for own betterment. He was looking after his own interests. He saw himself as the good, reliable, steady stalwart of his father. If he was a bird he would have been seen openly preening his feathers in the sun for all to see and thinking to himself, "What a good bird am I." While his brother was away he developed a haughty air of self-righteousness whenever his father mentioned his brother's name.

He was returning home after inspecting the distant fields of the estate when he heard music and merriment. Something was happening of which he knew nothing. Hurrying to find out, he met a servant bringing him the news of his brother's return. He became furious in jealous anger that his wastrel brother was being feted with a party. Even the fatted calf being kept for the next festival occasion had been killed. His hostility continued to ferment as he waited outside the house refusing to enter.

His father, a kindly loving man came out to soothe him and persuade him to come in and welcome his brother. The father had forgiven his wayward brother and desired that his elder son should do the same. The refusal to offer his brother forgiveness and welcome him back home left him outside antagonistic, annoyed and extremely displeased over his father's action and his disgraced brother's return. Pride and unwillingness to forgive kept piling on further fuel to the fire of his animosity toward his brother and his father. He paced up and down outside like a raging bull wanting to go on a rampage and vent his anger against his brother. A person, who refuses to forgive or consider forgiveness, ultimately, will find themselves on the outside filled with resentment and missing out on much of the good, joyous and peaceful opportunities life affords.

Character 8 – The Small Debtor

This poor man should not have been in the story. He was a typical battler whose life had not been easy. To help the family out of a difficulty, he borrowed a paltry sum from the high officer in the King's hierarchy. The officer who had been forgiven the fortune refused to forgive the small mortgage and demanded full payment and when it was not forthcoming threw him into gaol.

The repercussions of this malicious act had far reaching ramifications. Not only did the man have to languish in a squalid gaol, his family virtually became paupers because the breadwinner was in gaol. It is not only the unforgiven person who suffers but others associated with him. Also, the sadistic satisfaction received from exacting the penalty further sours and corrupts the spirit of the one who refused to forgive.

Caught In The Web of Unforgiveness

Here, we see the in these two characters the result of third parties caught in the web of forgiveness and unforgiveness. The father set the example of generosity in forgiveness after all he was the one who should have been offended and hurt by his younger son's self-destructive behavior. The elder brother refusal to forgive and welcome home his brother and bequeathed to him a spirit of animosity which maims a person's spirit so that a remedy is persistently refused.

In the case of the small debtor, he and his family had to suffer because the generosity of forgiveness was not passed on. The same consequences apply to the ungrateful servant as to the elder brother. Their future happiness was in jeopardy because of the unforgiving spirit. They finished their lives, unsociable, unloving and unlovable people when it all could have been so different.

From these three stories, we are compelled to consider the fruits of forgiving and receiving forgiveness.

What is Forgiveness

These three parables of Jewish origin have one principal theme – "Forgiveness." Each of these eight characters, in the parable, was involved in ways people in the present day may similarly be involved with situations of forgiveness and unforgiveness.

Lives are healed and made whole by the offer and acceptance of forgiveness. Without it they flounder in mediocrity, grief, sadness and loneliness. Comparable situations to these are likely to be met in pastoral ministry to individuals, families and communities.

Therefore we must ask, "What is forgiveness and what are the conditions for giving and receiving forgiveness?"

Forgiveness is a *voluntary gift.* The word voluntary should be underscored. A parent who tells her son that he should forgive a bully who has bloodied his nose and obeys his mother is not forgiveness. It is just a mouthful of words without meaning. The hurt emotional and physical stresses are still felt and the anger is still raging in the child's mind and heart. A person cannot be ordered to forgive another. If we look at the three authoritarian figures in our parables they did not have to offer forgiveness. The purpose of offering forgiveness to the exiled son was to lift him out of his misery and restore him hack to the family home. The forgiveness, offered the selfish son, restored him from servitude and squalor to respectability. The intent of abolishing that huge debt was to enable the lifting of a huge burden of shame, tension and stress from the ungrateful official's mind and to bring peace and stability back into his household. In each case it was compassion that reached out its arm of forgiveness to them.

Genuine forgiveness flows from a heart that has been wronged or hurt and yet is able to still have compassion for the one who has offended them so deeply. The forgiving one does not usually seek to gain materially or to receive accolades for their act. They anticipate the possibility of a restored relationship, harmony or an easing of tensions over what has happened. Forgiveness is a selfless act, voluntarily offered as a peace restoring offer.

Forgiveness *must arise out of our realization that we too are human.* To accept our own proneness to inflict physical and emotional hurt upon others is essential for true forgiveness. Often, the forgiving person is a person who has been hurt, injured, abused, maimed, dishonored, ridiculed, insulted, slandered or had material or personal losses in one form or another performed by other members of society against them at various times. That includes all of us.   Before forgiveness can be considered, the vision must rise above all the pummeling of the present stressful situation and admit that there have been and will be occasions when they must acknowledge responsibility for similar actions themselves. That is human nature.

The elder son in Jesus' parable was unable to offer forgiveness because he had not wasted his father's inheritance like his brother. This elder son could not see himself as being so prodigal and sinful. He also was jealous and resentful that his father had organized a welcome home celebration. Forgiveness is not forgiveness unless it is *offered with a degree of personal humility.*   Offered in a spirit of condescension it cannot be genuine forgiveness. Basically, we are little different from each other. We can never boast that with our underlying natures and being placed in similar circumstances and comparable stress we would not behave in the same offensive way. No one can claim to be perfect in all they do and say. By accepting that that is the case, then any forgiveness proffered will not have any air of superiority.

Forgiveness is *unconditional.* A parent who offers forgiveness in one breath and follows it with, "If you return to my house you will live according to my rules", has no real spirit of forgiveness. That is conditional forgiveness, which only reemphasizes the cause of the initial rebellious actions which caused the initial breach. A conditional forgiveness declares a continuing lack of trust. The victim has to show they are worthy of forgiveness by having to earn the right to be offered the forgiving spirit. In other words, acceptable behavior only is worthy of love and forgiveness. That is acceptable behavior in the eyes of the offered of the forgiveness not necessarily according to community standards. The authoritarian/subordination roles, the scenario of the previous offence being taken are maintained. *Conditional forgiveness is incomplete forgiveness.* On the other hand, the grateful recipient of forgiveness must show a desire to please the one from whom the forgiveness is received. Conditional forgiveness often places the forgiven under a never to be forgotten obligation.

A person commits an outrageous offence against the community. He is pilloried and publicly vilified so that the whole of society despises him. As the case comes to trial the background story of deprivation, physical and sexual abuse as a child is revealed. Because of his background from the wrong side of town, the police harassed him and made his life utterly miserable and so he cowered at the sight of them. Each day as the story unfolds in court the public anger turns to sympathy. His offence was understandable. Understanding can dispel blame and exonerate even antisocial behavior. Understanding of the background of antisocial behavior is not necessarily forgiveness. It can be helpful but it is not always necessarily so.

On the other hand, the grateful recipient of forgiveness must show a desire to please the one from whom the forgiveness is received.

Forgiveness is forgiveness when it covers inexcusable conduct. To understand the background and reasons for some sinful act or a series of ill and hurtful deeds is not forgiveness it may be called mercy. To find an excuse for such actions and receive the perpetrator back in to the family or society is accepting the reasons behind the action. To show mercy or to justify the hurtfulness provides a measure of healing of soured relationships and the restoration back into the community

Forgiveness is vastly different. The king in the first parable apparently had justifiable reasons for banishing his son. The son had no known justifiable reasons for his treachery against his father. It was inexplicable behavior. The king sent his officers to offer this son forgiveness for what people would have considered unpardonable behavior. The genuineness of the offer may also be assessed by the second effort to have a face to face meeting between the king and his son to cement the offer and acceptance of forgiveness.

Forgiveness Is a Self-healing Act

The victim of hurt is the one who offers forgiveness. The king was hurt by the son in exile. The father was hurt by the son who squandered the receipts of half of the estate. The generous king was hurt by the betrayed trust of his court official. Each of these gained a peace which healed the wounds of destroyed trust and hopes through sincerely offered forgiveness. Even where the forgiveness is not accepted, or even abused, the forgiver is able to rest in the knowledge that a no strings offer of forgiveness was made.

There is a true story of a thirteen year old girl who was repeatedly sexually abused by a priest. Torn between her respect for ordained clergy and the frightening introduction to sexual experience, she felt helpless and remained silent about it. She bottled her feelings deep within herself.

The psychological effects of the experiences and the repression of those feelings were dealt with in therapy some twenty plus years later. The anger, resentment and diminished self-respect were faced for the first time. After many months working with the therapist, she was able to write a non-judgmental letter to the priest outlining the damage and the dwarfing of her life he had caused over those twenty years. The letter contained an expression of forgiveness. The priest issued no reply nor sought forgiveness. Yet, that woman through that letter was opening the doors for him to respond, was able to feel as if she had been washed inside and outside cleansing her of her past sad experiences. She had her dignity and integrity restored. Her ability to relate to God and grow spiritually surged ahead. Forgiveness is an act of self-healing. The healing takes place when the anger and bitterness are released even though some scars may continue to show.

An article in Time magazine[14] said, "Inability to forgive is associated with persistent recrimination or dwelling on revenge while forgiving allows you to move on." Basically, forgiveness is an act of self-kindness.

Premature forgiveness takes place when it is merely a way to avoid unpleasant emotions or to please someone else, without dealing with the issue, and the consequences suffered, properly. It is frequently offered without a deep sincerity in order to bring about some semblance of peace while the grudge or resentment is allowed to remain. It might be called achieving a tolerated truce while the cause of the war still simmers.

A mediator, counselor, family member or friend may suggest the offer of forgiveness as a way forward for the victim. So long as the hurt remains there cannot be any real peaceful resolution to the situation or broken relationship. Hurt is hurt and must be openly admitted and dealt with before forgiveness should be considered. Forgive and forget is often urged upon the offended person. Something that has hurt deeply cannot be forgotten. It is only when it is genuinely and meaningfully forgiven can the effect of the hurt be minimized, inactivated or painlessly lived with. Where forgiveness is prematurely or immaturely offered, the pain is still carried. To try to forget in most cases is to repress the feelings which can have deep repercussions on the persons psyche and observable personality. To try to forget by offering premature forgiveness is to encase the problem more firmly in the sufferer's mind, preventing any possible release from the offence's repercussions.

Forgiveness and Reconciliation

Except for a few hermits and spiritual recluses we live in close intimacy in a family and/or a community. All of us are individuals whose view and perceptions on life differ. We have differing preferences. We go about

---

[14] Time Magazine dated 17th January, 2005 p.49.

our tasks of living by doing many things differently from others around us. Some of our differences may annoy or irritate our neighbors and colleagues. Generally, we are reasonably conciliatory and avoid disharmony by trying to accommodate others' idiosyncrasies.

However, there are times when our patience and intolerance become exhausted. Or another associate is deliberately and maliciously selfish or inconsiderately self-promoting. Such actions cause conflict, resentment, and physical or psychological I damage to ourselves and others. We are all prone to do it and are guilty of doing it from time to time as well as being on the receiving end of such anti-social behavior.

When we are the ones thus negatively affected with our pride wounded and anger stirred, among other things, then the responsibility falls on us to seek some reconciliation. The other person can apologize and make reparations or restitution, if able, which we should accept and offer forgiveness. In such cases where the offending party does not apologize and the tension and friction continues to mount, it is our responsibility to take the initiative and offer to forgive. Forgiveness goes beyond toleration or tacit acceptance of the other person's weakness or personality difficulty. Tolerance often masks a resentment which when sorely tried may flare into regrettable retaliatory action. Not only are we hurt by the other's actions, but, also, by our own harboring of those continuing inner tensions. By such, we destroy our own dignity and integrity in our own eyes and the eyes of others even if it is only because of our carping criticism of the offender. Unforgiveness, if allowed to continue, will only further demean us.

> *Tolerance often masks a resentment which when sorely tried may flare into regrettable retaliatory action. Not only are we hurt by the other's actions.*

Should we expect forgiveness to lead to reconciliation?

If we take the three parables there was forgiveness on the part of the father king toward his exiled son but no reconciliation. The father and the selfish son were reconciled and we shall see later the steps which lead to the amicable reunion. In the third parable there was a disastrous failure by the recipient of the forgiveness only to have the proffered forgiveness rescinded. In the first and third parables the forgiven offenders were left unchanged in nature by the forgiveness.

Reconciliation or a reunion of relationships is not always possible in all cases where forgiveness is initiated. As we have pointed out, the one initiating the offer of forgiveness does experience a healing of spirit and a sense of fulfilled responsibility demanded by the situation. All three forgivers in our parables were able to rest in the knowledge of having justified their obligations even if there remained some regrets that it did not completely achieve its intended purpose. They were able to get on with their lives, leaving those episodes behind them.

> *Reconciliation or a reunion of relationships is not always possible in all cases where forgiveness is initiated.*

The father king in the first parable may be considered to have been following the Jesus principle of forgiving seventy times seven. He left the offer of forgiveness open so that his son may return and take up the offer and be reconciled.

It must be remembered that the past cannot be changed, not can there be a return to the status quo. Things said and done have affected opinions, trust and circumstances. It is also difficult to change the character of the victimizer, however genuine the forgiveness or whether there was any reconciliation or not. On odd occasions where the one who is in need of forgiveness has a close encounter with reality as in the prodigal son then change may be possible; this is more likely if that encounter includes Godly direction. Forgiveness is not able to change the results of the past but it is able, in some cases, to cause a rethink, before the victimizer contemplates, committing the same damaging behavior again.

Each person has a personality which has developed through life's experiences from the day of birth. There are some personalities which are always prone to clash and differ on many matters of common interests. An offender carries a chip on the shoulder about life and people. Where there has been a harmful confrontation and only where the ill-feelings have been dealt with, may forgiveness be offered and received by both parties which can result in reconciliation, with those shoulder chips dealt with and removed.

In situations, where the two people concerned tote a high risk of further hurtful personality clashes, there may be an alternative reaction. The mutual offering of forgiveness may have little or no effect. It is better if they forgive and go their separate ways, avoiding all places where they are likely to again be closely associated. For these, their personalities naturally clash and in all probability will continue to do so where they take a differing stance on any issue.

Reconciliation can only take place where there is reciprocal accepting and compassionate interaction. The facts causing the friction must be acknowledged by both parties. That there are some grounds for the truth in some of the accusations and counter-accusations must be admitted by both. When that is accepted and the understanding of how each other feels is sincerely appreciated then the process of reconciliation is able to proceed in earnest,

> *Reconciliation can only take place where there is reciprocal accepting and compassionate interaction.*

What must be avoided is, what I call, *contracted reconciliation*. That is when the issues have not been adequately dealt with, even though; forgiveness has been offered and accepted. They may have agreed not to raise the offending subject in each other' presence again or let it influence matters between them in the future. A pastoral carer must not become involved in trying to broker reconciliation where doubt and mistrust of each other continues. To try to get them to work together with sincere cooperation will be fraught with tension. Where this is the case, the relationship is not natural, free and open, and they appear to be treading on egg shells every time they meet or are involved in any discussion in a committee or elsewhere - mutual trust remains short circuited. It is wiser if they pursue their interests in different communities or are involved in different programs and associations.

Steps to Reconciliation

Of the three parables only in the second do we see true forgiveness and reconciliation. We have just mentioned the possibility of mutual interaction between the two parties. It must include a sincere willingness to forgive and a genuine desire to be forgiven. We note that the father was ever waiting and waiting to receive and forgive his son. However, the son, the one needing to be forgiven, had to take certain steps in order to receive the blessing of forgiveness.

Basically, we see four steps:
- Acceptance of the situation.
- Confession of foolishness and selfishness
- Repentance for the sin-ridden condition
- Readiness to face and accept the penalty.

Here was a selfish son that was in that "Woe is me" situation. His money had run out. His fair-weather friends had deserted him. Ragged and forlorn, he was ravenously hungry as he watched the pigs feeding on their swill. Even that vile mush seemed as tempting as a royal feast to the palace slave of yesteryear. He had descended to a nobody, swine herdsman with no home, no possessions, torn clothes, and no friends. Were there ever a more despised and wretched individual? This was his present situation in life; he first had to accept it.

In those lone times in the day and during the long sleepless hours of the night, with the lice, multiplying in his hair and the fleas from the pigs reminding him of his plight, he was compelled to confess to himself what a fool and idiot he was.

So many who have violated the moral and ethical laws of human living, at times, are able to recognize the foolishness of their reckless ways and how they have defied social and godly norms. Previously, they have ignored them; tried to cover up their

actions; blamed others; exaggerated the events to avoid responsibility or denied their implication by lying. So long as they continue to hide behind such deception they will never come to the point of confessing their self-indulgence and sinfulness against others and God. With confession, the totality of the inappropriateness of their life style is exposed.

However, it is not sufficient to confess or own up to the sinful, unholy life. It needs to be accompanied by repentance. Repentance involves change of heart and a determination to abandon the causes of the plight they are in. Confession is a head and verbal acknowledgment of it. Repentance involves resolution and action to change. It is thus more than head; it involves a determination to turn the life around by starting to follow the path that leads to right living; the type of life that will restore dignity and respect. None, whose job was to feed pigs, in those days, could expect to be respected by others. Repentance produces a new type of behavior, a different one from that which led to the pig sty.

However, it is not sufficient to confess or own up to the sinful, unholy life. It needs to be accompanied by repentance.

Genuine repentance is ready to accept the penalty for, make restitution or reparations for the consequences of the rebellious sinful life being abandoned. The prodigal son in his confession and repentance for his past living said that he would go to his father, confess his sinfulness and accept the penalty by becoming a servant in his father's house. The penalty he was willing to face was the loss of sonship and demotion to servant hood. In the reality check on his life, he saw that that was the most he could expect from his father. A repentant person has no grand notion of being promoted or restored in status because of the willingness to change.

In cases where the broken relationship or the offence inflicted suffering of one sort or another upon the victim, then, that damage has to be repaired. Where the victim has suffered financial hardship, then, the repentant one has to face the penalty of repaying the financial loss. The penalty may involve bearing the consequences of the wrongful acts committed.

Without the following of these steps, it is difficult for the forgiveness to be fully appropriated. Without confession and repentance, the exiled son was unable to accept the offered forgiveness. The king's official who accepted the forgiveness as an easy way out of his predicament showed no sign of remorse or repentance, so, he lost the privilege of being totally forgiven and so he languished in gaol. Only the prodigal son's experience of forgiveness and reinstatement within his father's house brings true peaceful forgiveness and resolution.

These may be three parables; yet, they clearly show God's method of dealing with sinful living and the means of being restored into God's blessing and being totally forgiven by both God and man.

Pastoral Intervention

Any ministry to a person who has been the victim of offensive words or actions requires some understanding of the above vagaries of forgiveness. Your ministry may or may not lead to reconciliation between the two parties. If it can lead to an offer of forgiveness, whether it is accepted or not, is the object of pastoral care in such cases. To try and press too hard for reconciliation may negate all your efforts and even alienate the person(s) with whom you are dealing. Always keep in mind that any act of forgiveness opens wide the spirit of the forgiver to healing and peace which comes from the heart of God himself. God has set the pattern of forgiveness though his willingness to free each and every human being from the power and guilt of sin no matter how heinous or trivial the erring may have been.

The role of the pastoral visitor is to encourage forgiveness to the victim against whom injustices have been committed. To offer forgiveness is to be released from the bondage of anger, bitterness, a critical spirit and the desire for spiteful retaliation. To lead a person to the point of forgiveness is to help restore peace into the heart of a very troubled person. It covers and helps to minimize the destructiveness of the sin that has been committed against them.

The offender may or may not be changed by the offer, whether it is accepted or not. It is possible to make a difference to the person's reaction to the past. The significance of the past is mellowed by the forgiving spirit. The practical repercussions may not be appreciably changed such as when it caused a death. Forgiveness may change how the victim of the abuser lets the past continue to affect him or her by removing much or only a little of the sting.

Forgiveness is able to bring a sense of release, absolution from any guilt over the affair, and a renewed confidence to relate with other people. A greater attitude of caution in dealing with people may remain. This may be good in that it maintains a greater awareness of possible further relationship breakdowns and thus act to such possibility. Where the victim has been gullible, caution may enable alertness to future manipulative ploys against them

In dealing with the victimizer or offender, the same slowly, slowly approach must be made as to the victim. The victim may accuse you of being too insensitive if you try to press for their action to forgive too soon. The offender may on the other hand charge you with interfering in something that is not your business. It must be remembered that the victimizer will be on the defensive almost as soon as they see you. They often cannot see that they have done anything wrong and that it was all as a result of the victim's attitude or behavior. They may not be able or willing to admit that they have erred in any way. It will take time to build up sufficient confidence in you before any objective look at the situation can be broached. That objective overview, if delicately handled, may bring about that initial acceptance of what actually happened and the real causes for it. From there, the steps to reconciliation may follow in order.

> *To interfere in a situation where two parties are bitter and antagonistic, it requires, as some would say, 'the wisdom of Solomon'.*

To interfere in a situation where two parties are bitter and antagonistic, it requires, as some would say, 'the wisdom of Solomon'. At times Solomon's wisdom may not be enough. That wisdom may be to back off because more trouble is being brewed by your untimely opening up the issue.

Pastoral care should not enter the courts of such situations without thorough personal spiritual preparation and have the deep inner conviction that you are on His mission and that He is your ever present advisor. The ultimate of pastoral care in such situations is, where possible, to leave both the victim and the victimizer reconciled with God and at peace with Him – the great exemplar of "Forgiveness".

CHAPTER 9

The Discerning Disabled

As a teenager, a young woman who was associated with our group was disabled from birth. She was born with cerebral palsy. She had virtually no use of any of her four limbs, all being twisted and deformed. Her face and speech were severely distorted. Her full brain function made her as mentally alert as any normal healthy person, yet, out of the wheel chair, she had to be carried everywhere. We included Miriam in any special meeting or event to which we could take her. We saw her as a valuable, loved and an integral member of the youth group. Once a month, we held our meetings in her home to which she made her valuable contributions. She often offered some pearls of wisdom and grace which was very sobering and meaningful for the group.

I could see the depth of character in her. Her realistic faith was in her God and Savior. My heart reached out to her. My faith at that age believed that whatever we sincerely and with unswerving faith asked of God He would do. That was if it was not a selfish prayer for our own benefit and so I prayed for the full use of her body to be gained. Of course that healing did not take place. It was not for lack of faith on my part. Since then Paul's thorn in the flesh and his testimony to the Phillipian church that he knew what it was to have sufficient and what it was to be facing hardship and deprivation has enriched my understanding of such situations. He was able to testify that he had the strength given by Christ to be contented whatever his condition. (Phil. 4:12-13). Miriam, I believe, exemplified Paul's position even though her perpetual handicaps seemed to outweigh Paul's hardships. Through her twisted body, her mind and spirit radiated and confirmed in modern times what faith and intimacy in the living God can do.

Miriam's life taught me that our spirit and its relationship with God are more important than a full functioning, physical body. This has been repeatedly confirmed in my ministry to hospital patients with physical and mental disabilities.

The word disabled, used in its broader sense, to the physically and mentally disabled, may include the spiritually and socially disabled. For this exercise, we shall concentrate on physical and mental disability.

What Is Disability?

In order for pastoral care to be effective as possible, the carer must keep him or her informed of contemporary man's needs-particularly those who are suffering from some form of disability. To visit a person for the first time, who has shaking hands and slurred speech, it may be assumed that the person is intoxicated. The person may be in the early stages of motor neuron disease, in which the person's nervous system is breaking down or is recovering from meningitis, Parkinson's Disease, a stroke or some such illness of the nervous system, affecting speech and limbs. Their intellectual function may be sharp and keen and they are able to discern any indication the carer gives of disdain or wrong assessment. The carer needs to be aware of the types of disabilities and the nature of their presentation. In some cases, this may be further elucidated by the person visited as they often desire to air the nature of their condition.

In 1980 the World Health Organization published a document entitled, "International Classification of Impairments, Disabilities and Handicaps." Those three categories would be a good place to start to understand human body and mental dysfunction.

Impairment is any loss or abnormality of psychological, physiological or anatomical structure or function.

Disablement is any restriction or lack (resulting from an impairment) of ability to perform any activity in a manner or way considered normal for human beings.

Handicap is a disadvantage for a given individual resulting from impairment or disability that limits or prevents the fulfillment of a role that is normal (depending on age, sex, social and cultural factors) for the individual. Impairment, as defined, may be physical, or psychological. A *physical impairment* may be the result of the malfunction, deformity, or removal of an organ or limb which does not allow the body to fully function as a normal human being. In the case of Miriam it was a physical impairment caused by congenital brain damage which partially paralyzed her limbs and affected her ability to speak normally.

Psychological impairment of a person is any condition which affects their normal intellectual abilities for their age, such as being unable to make rational assessments of any given situation or take appropriate actions for their age. Miriam had full mental discernment and logical reasoning.

The impairment of a person may be both physical and psychological. The loss of any one of the physical sensory functions such as sight, hearing, touch, smell and speech severely incapacitate a person's ability to function normally. Although, with medical and mechanical aids, the affects may be minimized by using spectacles, hearing aids, cochlea implants, prostheses etc. Down's syndrome children may be born with some physical or some defect of an organ in addition to some weakened mental function. They, however, can have a sharp wit and humor and are exceptionally affectionate. Persons with both physical and psychological impairments are said to have multiple malfunctions. Where intellectual impairment combines with physical disorders, pastoral workers will need to prepare themselves with some research on intellectual sub-normality.

Disability is any form of functional loss caused by physical or psychological impairment. As such the nature and severity of functional loss varies from person to person. Disability may affect people in various ways of normal functioning. The most obvious is the loss of a limb, loss of sight, muscle wastage of a limb, paralysis or partial paralysis of a limb, hearing or speech difficulties, any of which may impede their ability to move independently without instrument or medical aids. That is, the person's mobility is affected and they cannot carry out normal human activity for their age,

A disabled person is usually unable to be engaged in full time employment outside the home, except in specially designed places of work to aid their disability or in Sheltered Workshops. Some disabled people are unable to care for their personal hygiene, washing and grooming. Their ability for independent self care is severely limited. When it comes to doing ordinary household chores, their limitations are noticeable. Tasks such as making beds, ironing, cooking and shopping are often not able to be performed without some aid.

Handicap –The popular use of the word handicapped has been applied to any disabled person. In modern parlance, handicap should not be used interchangeably with disablement i.e. a handicapped person is disabled but a person disabled may not be handicapped. A handicapped person is one whose social life and skills are disadvantaged. Some cerebrally disabled persons have been able to capitalize on their impairments. I know of at least two cerebrally palsied comedians who have gained international reputations as standup comedians. Socially they are acclaimed and associate and interact with people better than a large percentage of people without any impairment.

The Causes of Impairment and Disability.

There are many causes of impairment and disability. For ease of understanding we shall place them in three categories: Congenital, Sudden Onset and Gradual Onset.

Congenital Disabilities

As the name suggests, they are conditions which develop in the womb, and are generally evident immediately after delivery, unless detected earlier in the ultra-sounds. In some cases, defective hearing and sight may not be detected till later and sometimes not until they attend school. In some hospital settings, a pediatrician and not the obstetrician will examine the infant to detect if there is any impairment which needs to be watched and followed up before the babe is released from hospital.

Congenital conditions can affect any part of the body. Some cardiac conditions require corrective surgery within hours of the birth or as soon as possible after birth. One of the most notable defects is in respiration. This may be the result of respiratory weakness, smoking during the pregnancy etc. Stress, tension, or some physical trauma such as asthma the mother went through during the pregnancy can have serious affects upon the fetus. Cerebral palsy, cystic fibrosis, spina bifida, Down's syndrome, some epilepsy, congenital blindness, or neural damage affecting limbs may be the result of a condition developed after conception. Some of the sources of the problem may be a genetic abnormality in either one or both the parental genes. These physical impairments may later produce psychological impairment when their physical difference interferes with their socialization. There are times when long and stressful deliveries can so stress the fetus so that oxygen supply to the brain is interfered with causing intellectual impairment to be revealed later. As the child begins to develop, a congenitally impaired child grows up knowing no other condition yet becomes aware that they are different from other children and may have to attend special schools. Many an impaired child becomes aware of the difference by being made fun of by other children or being rejected by other children and adults. Many a marriage has been torn apart by the birth of a congenitally deformed child. The father has insufficient emotional stability to deal with a mal-formed offspring. He may ignorantly blame some fault in his manhood for such an outcome.

Terry was born with a receding extra high forehead, bulging eyes and a receding jaw line. The last defect threatened to shut off his windpipe. The father totally rejected the child. He never visited him in hospital. When allowed out of the hospital for a Sunday afternoon drive, the father would drive the mother and child to a park. Leave them at the far gate and meet them at the other end of the park when it was time to return to the hospital.

The father moved in with another woman twelve months after the birth. At sixteen months a major decision about reconstruction surgery had to be made. It required three different surgical specialists and an operation which had never been attempted in the world before. The outcome of which was very uncertain. It was an enormous responsibility to place on the mother. The father would not see the doctor. As the Chaplain, I accompanied and supported her when she went to the Director of Surgery to discuss the procedure and make the decision. The surgery was a success but the weakened immune system of the child led to pneumonia causing the child's death three weeks later.

Many fathers cannot accept that their child's condition is congenital impairment. Some perhaps feel responsible for the condition. Others, falsely, see it as a reflection on their masculine virility. The pastoral carer should be alert for any signs of such family dynamics when visiting such a family.

Sudden Onset

Sudden onset of impairment raises the spectrum of many origins for such impairment leading to serious disabilities. The ones that immediately spring to mind are cases of accidents of all kinds: road, sporting, boating, drowning, falls, drug overdoses etc. The person has been fit, healthy, ambitious and socially popular then suddenly a misadventure of one sort or another occurs so that their active life abruptly ceases and they lay in hospital with hospital staff trying to restore mobility, agility, encourage speech and even mental or other sensory functions.

For them it is a sudden reversal of fortunes. It is a sudden halt to the only type of living they had known. Their future dreams, aspirations, way of life are all abruptly broken. It brings the emotional response similar to a death, for that it what it is – a death to a way of life. They are stunned, disbelieving and full of unrealistic hopes which do not allow for the truth of the doctor's prognosis to be accepted. Moreover, they are angry over the cause of the change, blaming others, exonerating themselves, or remorsefully guilty over their own carelessness, stupidity, and even stubbornness.

They shed tears over the future. How will they manage? Who will look after them? How will they survive financially? Will they be able to find suitable employment? These are some of the questions that distress them in the post-accident period.

Elsewhere, it has been mentioned of a budding Olympic hopeful whose lower leg was severed when he slipped between the station platform and an incoming train. He repeatedly talked of suicide as he did not see his planned future being fulfilled. At first, he rejected my suggestion of the possibility of competing in the Para-Olympics. His life was finished, so he thought. He scoffed at the repeated suggestion. However, the seed thoughts of the Para-Olympics sunk into his subconscious to be resurrected after leaving the hospital and continuing with his physiotherapy and rehabilitation. He put his whole effort into salvaging as much as he could of his life. He eventually was successful at the Para-Olympics winning gold in the wheelchair discus event. In one respect, through his impairment he achieved more than he might have done otherwise. The competition for a place in the national team for the normal Olympics was strong and his chances were slim.

I was involved in an emergency room where up to six bicycle accidents per week were admitted. Often, the youthful cyclists were not wearing helmets. In most cases, the head injuries were serious, resulting in death or permanent brain damage with some remaining in a vegetative state.

The ones that immediately spring to mind are cases of accidents of all kinds: road, sporting, boating

Personally, the most heartbreaking

experience is to enter the adolescent ward of the annex of a Pediatric hospital away from the main campus. All the patients were in their late teens. All lay in a fetal position with no brain responsiveness and being tube fed. Each of these ten or so patients had been in this vegetative state after near drowning accidents when they were four or five years of age. Their families had long since ceased visiting them because they were never recognized by their child nor was any communication possible. The child was never aware of anyone being present. For the parents, a visit only would afford irremediable personal pain and regret over a life that might have been. Some parents in such situations also bear a load of guilt for not providing sufficient supervision to avoid the accident.

Accidents frequently result in sudden onsets of disability and handicaps. These are not the only ways impairment occurs. There are diseases which result in degenerative conditions of the organs or neurological function. These may cause the curtailment of certain more strenuous activities and perhaps develop into more serious disability.

Cardio-vascular accidents may include the flaking off of plaque from the arteries leading to the heart and brain. These form blockages leading to heart attacks and strokes. The latter may cause the dying of some of the brain cells by the stopping of the flow of the blood to those cells. Depending upon the brain cells thus affected, it results in the malfunction of the nervous system which may partially paralyze certain parts of the body. Cells on the right side of the brain control left-sided function and the left sided brain damage cause right sided paralysis and speech impediment. There can be some restoration of the function up to two months following the cardio-vascular accident, depending upon the degree of healing possible in the brain. Rehabilitation therapy in some cases may help recover some physical activity and some speech improvement.

The sudden deprivation of the blood supply to the brain is called an infarct. The blockage is caused by embolism or thrombosis (blood clots), fat globules or gas bubbles variably called a cardio-vascular thrombic-embolic accident, Transient Ischemic Attack (TIA) or stroke.

Brain tumors also may cause a sudden onset of impairment. Depending on their location in the brain, brain tumors may be controlled by chemotherapy, radiotherapy or surgery. A tumor behind the eye can cause loss of vision. Other brain tumors can result in personality change, paralysis of part of the body, thinking and speech ability as well as resulting in a vegetative state. Other body tumors can cause similar damage to the parts of the body according to their location.

A nine year old boy playing hockey was struck hard by a hockey ball just above his knee. Two years later he was diagnosed with a tumor where he was struck by the ball. A few months later it was spreading so fast that the leg had to be amputated at the top of the thigh. Tumors in other areas may have disabling consequences. Lung cancer, renal cancer and liver cancer may mean that these organs cannot function fully and therefore restricts the patient' ability to fully participate in life as they once did.

Sudden onset of disability may arise from a variety of sources.

Gradual Onset

Deterioration of the ability of various parts of the body to function normally is often slow, sometimes due to the aging process. Neurological diseases such as multiple sclerosis, muscular dystrophy or motor neuron disease, also may be seen in younger adults and can develop until wheelchair bound or confined to bed requiring total care. In such cases, their intellectual ability remains unaffected and so they feel themselves trapped inside their physically inactive body. A young nurse educator when lecturing found she was dropping her whiteboard pen whilst she was writing. It was the first signs of her multiply sclerosis. She was in her late twenties.

The opposite of those neurological conditions are that of dementia and Alzheimer's which may show first signs in mid-life. In dementia the thinking capacity becomes addled. Physically they may be fit and capable for their age. The mental deterioration gradually gets worse until they require twenty four hour observation or care. Some dementia patients may become aggressive when efforts are made to restrain their inappropriate behavior

There are progressive disabilities due to the worsening of the condition of various organs of the body to function. Diseases such as tuberculosis, tobacco smoking, asbestosis and other respiratory problems so debilitate and weaken the body that they become severely handicapped. Sugar diabetes often caused by heart condition, obesity, fatty foods and poor nutrition, if uncontrolled, does more than reduce activity; it can also cause damage to the circulation of blood to the extremities of the limbs causing gangrene requiring limb amputations.

There are joint problems which retard mobility and flexibility of a person's movement. The most obvious of these, which can affect younger people although they are more prevalent in the later years, are arthritis and rheumatism. Sports injuries and frequent, hard, rough jarring of the joints are conducive for the development of arthritis. Wrong posture and unwise repetitious use of hips and lower limbs can place strain and wear on the joints, requiring replacement of hips and knees. I knew of one International Rugby League player of the 1920's, who, twenty years later, walked with great difficulty and his other joints and limbs were so painful that he was constantly on painkillers. Similar familiar stories are told of modern sports achievers requiring knee replacements, shoulder surgery, painkillers in joints before playing etc. Impairment, disability and handicap can be traced to so many causes resulting in pain and loss of function in different parts of the body. Each sufferer reacts in different ways and endures their disablement differently, with differing impacts on their personality and ways of relating. The person making a pastoral visit must be alert to some of the causes and reaction of patients to physical impairment.

The Disabled's Despair

Richie was a sixteen year old football player in his High School's team. He was popular with the players as well as his many female fans. His recent illness had been diagnosed as cancer of the kidneys. It was suspected that it may have been caused by a football injury in his junior years. On his admission to hospital, where he had gone to have one of the kidneys removed, he was surrounded each afternoon and evening by his many admirers. As his stay in hospital was prolonged and the realization dawned that he would not play football again, there was an appreciable drop in the number of visitors. By the third week, there were only two or three of his genuine friends coming to visit him. Not one of the girls came near him.

Richie was now impaired. He was not nor ever would be again the physical person he was before. So the interest in him waned largely because they did not know what to say to him and that there could not be any normal teenage interaction with him. The silences were embarrassing for all. Talk of football and school antics only brought sullen responses. Ritchie felt rejected and abandoned. As the truth of his future condition, which he had been denying, sank in, he became further depressed. This depression turned to despair as he noticed the absence of his friends. Richie died eighteen months later from a heart attack. One specialist in a clinical meeting suggested that Ritchie's reaction to his disablement and the desertion of his friends might have brought on the heart condition. Others might conclude that it was a psychosomatic death.

Richie is an extreme case of the reaction to impairment. It should alert the visitor that any visit to the recently disabled may be complicated and carry with it significant responsibility. It does highlight some of the psychological impositions that impairment makes.

The visitors also stopped coming because they could see Ritchie's frustration at not being able to participate in their banter and his humiliation at being in his pajamas and in bed feeling useless and of no consequence to anyone. He spent hours each day comparing his present condition to what it was six months earlier, what it might have been and what it possibly will be. A disabled person usually has plenty of time to reflect and anticipate the horrors of entrapment in a disabled body,

As has already been illustrated, a father disowned his congenitally deformed son. Ritchie's father had the same reaction. When a member of the family has an impairment of any sort, it affects the whole family dynamics in the way they relate to each other in the new circumstances. Other siblings are often neglected or have to put in extra effort into assisting in the things about the home and in the care of the incapacitated family member. This often builds up feelings of resentment and of being a less loved member of the family. The extra responsibilities may compel the need to reduce some of their normal social opportunities which again may result in the weakening of the sibling's important friendships because they cannot attend certain activities. In so many cases, I have experienced that a husband or father find it difficult to handle that a member of the family, wife or offspring, is permanently handicapped. When this happens, the marriage has little chance of maintaining warmth and passion and may end in separation and divorce, further complicating the situation. The one impaired is likely to take up a burden of guilt over the marriage break down.

Arthur had a disabling condition which was a gradual deterioration. The early symptoms of tiredness, lethargy and lack of concentration were treated with the usual tonics and nutritional advice. The accompanying headaches were relieved by painkillers. Scans were ordered and showed the cause to be a brain tumor. For more than twelve months he had been attending doctors. In that time, the tumor had developed so much that risky surgery was necessary. Radiotherapy shrunk the tumor to make surgery less dangerous. The operation while successful left him with a partial paralysis down the right side.

Following his diagnosis, Arthur became very resentful that his condition had not been detected earlier. He was abusive and very aggressive to all medical staff. He could not bring himself to trust anything that a doctor said to him. When he realized after the operation that he had a permanent disability he threatened to sue the medical practitioner for negligence.

Before the surgery, he held an important executive position which predictably determined his reactions. He was used to being in charge and issuing orders. Now he had to respect the word of others and obey instructions. Not only was his ability to function normally destroyed but his whole self-image was shattered. He was a shadow of his former self. From being a fiercely aggressive executive, he was reduced in stature to being dependent on others for some of his daily needs. Arthur remained an ungrateful recipient of all the assistance that was offered him and refused to see his former business colleagues. For years, he remained a morose, cantankerous person for whom family and professional persons continued faithfully to attend to his needs. Dealing with him required considerable patience even by his wife who would have gladly walked away from him.

Arthur's reaction was the opposite of George, whose stroke left him with partial paralysis restricting his mobility, causing him to have difficulty in saying the right word. He knew what he wanted to say but the right word would just not come out. The frustration of being so embarrassed by this, George's humiliation forced him to repress his emotions, particularly his anger, and become non-communicative with friends outside the family. The family had great difficulty in trying to persuade him to go out for a drive in the country in case they met someone they knew. His mono-syllabic responses at attempted conversation left the family also emotionally disturbed.

In looking at the cases of Ritchie whose reaction to his disability possibly led to an unexpected premature death, Arthur who became aggressive and intolerant of all others, and George, who, with his repressed emotions, became docile, withdrawn and unsociable, we are forced to ask ourselves the question, "Why these three different types of reaction?"

The reason for these reactions is basically the same; each one was grieving over the loss of part of their true selves. A part of them and their persona had died never to be recovered. Ritchie lost his kidney and his sporting ambitions, Arthur his authority, independence and leadership, and George his speech and ability to converse and socialize, each responded to their losses according to their personal perception of the magnitude of their deprivation and their ability to cope. Their grief in each case was as devastating as their disability. The pastoral carer must recognize the grief dynamics in visiting a handicapped person, particularly a newly disabled person. The emotional disturbance, which is affecting relatives and friends also, should not be overlooked.

Pastoral Intervention

The pastoral visitor should not be overwhelmed by the complexity of the problems that may be encountered in meeting the needs of the physically or intellectually impaired if he or she has undertaken some supervised pastoral training.

The Appraisal

Many people in meeting the disabled approach them with a sense of pity in its most objectionable, patronizing context. The Samaritan saw a temporarily disabled person on the road. Jesus said he had pity or compassion on him and took action providing first-aid and then taking him to a place where he would get further help to heal his wounds. It was not a condescending pity nor an obligated pity but a genuine desire to help and restore the victim to wholeness.

As he looked at that man with physical impairment on the road, he saw not a poor wretch who had been beaten and robbed. He looked upon a fellow human being with potential if cared for practically, sensitively and encouragingly. He looked upon a person like himself. Here was a person with the possibilities for restoration to some meaningful life. So the pastoral carer should view the disabled. We, as teenagers, saw in Miriam a person who was able to make a valuable contribution to our group in spite of her twisted body, face and distorted speech. I am grateful to God for that early encounter with handicapped Miriam.

It must be remembered that a disabled person's needs are constantly changing. Any pastoral intervention depends upon the stage of the disability, (recent or long term), the degree of dependency and the extent to which the grief has been confronted. No matter how long or how recently you have known the patient being visited, and impairment will have brought changes to his or her attitude and outlook on life. It has often happened that a once church-friendly person has become bitter and angry toward God because of the physical affliction. A careful, sensitive appraisal of the person's state and mental attitude to the situation must be made if an effective, supportive pastoral ministry is to be meaningful to the person. Remember, it is the spirit of the person that is the real person and not wholeness of bodily looks or function.

The offering of pastoral care to such people may include:
- Being there as a companion
- Identifying positive possibilities
- Assistance in developing more independence
- Practical support - such as providing or organizing transport
- Dealing with intellectual and theological issues
- Long term interest and care
- Creating opportunities for socialization and fellowship
- To enable the incapacitated person to live as rich and full a life as possible

Being a Companion

It has been said that no man is an island and that everyman is a piece of the continent and part of the main land. Ministry to the disabled should be constantly reminding us of this. Often, the church and society view the disabled as islands separated from the mainstream of life. They are different. We treat them differently because they cannot do all the things we can do and they cannot get to the places the rest of us can. It is too difficult to include them in certain programs as they will slow us down. So, again and again, the disabled are not included and deliberately not invited for one reason of inconvenience or another. Frequently, we who are able bodied cause or further cause them to feel an isolated island and not part of the main stream of society. We occasionally row across river that separates them from the rest of society to say hello to let them know that they are not entirely forgotten.

In the case of Miriam, she was included in much of our social activities. On social nights, we felt elated to see her laughing in her own way at some of our youthful antics. When we went to the beach, she sat on the sand as part of the group. We provided for her youthful companionship in what would have been a very isolated life.

In any ministry of care to the disabled the first consideration is that the visit should provide companionship for a person who is unable to be as active as normal people. Companionship creates a feeling of belonging, of being accepted and of being a human who is valued by a friend(s).

One of the thoughts constantly being emphasized by society upon the handicapped is that they are different and should be treated differently. Certainly, their ability to function in life is abnormal. The insensitivity of many humans toward the impaired, whether psychological or physical, is that they are less than human because of the bodily weakness. The genuine pastoral person is able to show true acceptance, appreciate their company and conduct an unembarrassed normal conversation.

Encourage Deeper Conversation

These words -unembarrassed and normal- are keywords when in the company of the impaired. So frequently, they find people stand or sit with them not knowing what to say. Even the greeting, "How are you?" stick in their throats in case they hear a tale of woe, of aches and pains, or of the difficulties of being handicapped. They do not expect to have a normal conversation. Except for the mentally impaired, their minds are normal. They listen to the radio, watch TV and read newspapers and magazines. Most are perfectly capable of conducting a normal conversation. They too have special interests, hobbies and perhaps may be employed part time or full time, about which they are able to express themselves.

A caller from the church may have additional offerings to make. A pastoral person should be seen as one who has qualities of truthfulness, reliability, keeps confidences, discernment, understanding, spiritual wisdom and has a good listening ear. With these gifts, the one being visited may be encouraged to open up, or be drawn out to verbalize on matters that may be of concern to them or have been affecting them personally and in their relating with others, particularly the church and its attitude. Another may have passed some hurtful patronizing remark which they have been bottling up and want to talk it out or someone has been avoiding them. More importantly, they may be harboring strong negative feelings about their condition or are even inwardly accusing God of being malicious, unfeeling and unloving.

Realizing that the mind and situation of the disabled person may differ from visit to visit, the carer, as has already been mentioned, should first of all try to discern the attitude and mood of the person on each visit. Any indifference toward you as a church visitor may be because of some negative experience with a church member. They may be generally exasperated with their condition or angry because God hasn't been answering their prayers.

If possible, the carer should be unobtrusively trying to elicit the expression of these wounded feelings that they are trying to bury or are fuming over. Most handicapped people need to be able to engage in deeper conversation than the weather and topical newspaper items.

Identifying Positive Possibilities

As a child, he contracted meningitis. This left him with a degree of mental retardation. His schooling was abruptly ended. Now, some two decades later, he has difficulty in reading and writing; otherwise his body functions are normal. Since his mother's death he has been accommodated in a hostel situation where all his needs are catered for, including room-cleaning, laundry and meals. He has a somewhat naïve yet willing spirit. He listens to radio and TV news and latches onto crime which troubles him greatly.

If he was left to himself, he would annoy the other residents morning, noon, and night. He likes to know everything that is happening around the place and dwells on the negative. Minor episodes are reported as major dramas. This causes him to be solicitous for the personal welfare and possessions of his neighbors warning them constantly to be wary and careful. He has a very willing and caring spirit. It is that spirit which was able to be used to develop opportunities for his usefulness and thus build up his self-esteem and give him the knowledge that he had a useful place in society. The administration encouraged him to take out the garbage bins and clear the waste bins from the kitchen. This led to him running errands for the office staff. When there is a concert or other function in the hall he is asked to assist in setting out the chairs, tables etc, and to put them away. On the day of the fete he is a very busy man doing all sorts of tasks. He then was officially given a badge as a volunteer and each year, at the Christmas party, he is acknowledged for his work as a volunteer. He has a sense of pride in himself as a volunteer and as a good helper.

He is extremely happy in this environment. It is a church institution with a pastoral heart. He is not seen as an ordinary resident. They have been able to see, in this man now in his fifties, his special needs and saw the positive possibilities of his childlike willingness. Every word of appreciation and thanks for his help is as good for him as a bucket of ice cream to a small child. It provides him with the incentive to be faithful to his allotted tasks and he always puts his best effort into what he does. The pastoral spirit saw in him positive possibilities. Without these his life would be lived in the spirit of a morbid depression of uselessness, seeing only the negative and being paranoid about all that happens around him. Dwelling on such, day in and day out would create objections from his fellow residents because of his annoying intrusions into their lives with such concerns.

Developing Independence

Sympathy and compassion can be overzealous and in doing so counter the very helpful intentions of providing companionship and generating conversation. A well meaning visitor can see a handicapped person struggling to do some simple thing about the house or group; they rush to assist them out of the kindness of their heart. There is a saying, 'without pain there is no gain'. This is a valuable word to constantly have in mind when in the company of the disabled.

It is important for their self-esteem and convenience that a person who has a significant loss of bodily function and mobility is able to do as much for themselves (however difficult), as possible. We may see such a one struggle and at times wince as they try to go beyond their own accomplishments since the incapacitation. It is like a war to be won for them. They are at war with their condition and each new achievement is a battle won. They will continue to struggle and repeat the process until the task or whatever they are trying to do is done and their confidence to improve next time is strengthened. Where you see such determination it should be encouraged. There will be some things that are simply too difficult and a helping hand might be appreciated. Sensitivity and awareness to promote independence or offer assistance must be ever discerning. For the disabled person to do something new for themselves is a sense of achievement and victory. To encourage them in other situations to try something more difficult also shows your confidence in them that they can do it. The more they can do for themselves the better.

A specialist teacher on 'Stewardship' was brought out, from the United States, by the National Christian Council of India. He told of an experience he had in the Philippines. A missionary couple employed a household help who lived on the mission compound and was dependent upon the missionaries for most of her needs. When it came to Sunday they gave her offering to put in the plate. The stewardship teaching urged that the next Sunday they should make a special effort and give a thank offering. The dutiful

> *It is important for their self-esteem and convenience that a person who has a significant loss of bodily function and mobility is able to do as much for themselves.*

missionary gave this home help a considerably larger amount as her offering. This missionary's worker sought out the Stewardship teacher who was staying in the home and wept volubly. Through her tears she said, "They won't even let me give my own offering to the Lord."

Those well meaning missionaries were stripping their worker of her independence and denying her the opportunity of the joy of giving for herself as well as deciding for herself how much she should give. They had forgotten Jesus' observation of the woman who gave her mite into the temple treasury

Many pastoral people treat a disabled person in the same way, rushing in to help them when they see that they cannot perform the task as well as themselves. I have seen a disabled person get up to pour a glass of juice to serve their guest only to have the jug snatched from their hands and the visitor do the pouring for those present - a repeat of that missionary scenario.

Cindy, the partially paralyzed person who had poured drinks on many occasions previously was further made to feel useless and redundant. Cindy was deeply hurt and inwardly cried, "They won't even let me pour a glass of water."   The incident highlighted her physical impairment and the regard this person had of her.

One of the most helpful things a pastoral person can do is, where appropriate, to promote a spirit of independence as much as possible. It may be painful to watch them try to do something. When they achieve something difficult, a word of praise is encouraging. If something arises to be done that it may cause the person some difficulty, awkwardness and even pain to do it then let them to do it if they desire to attempt it. Any achievement is another victory for them, more expertise is gained in doing what has been achieved, and above all their spirit has been lifted. In these cases, it is best for the carer to take the more passive role. The handicapped is then seen to be an achiever.

Offering Practical Support

There are some things a disabled person cannot do on their own. Some handicapped people are able to drive specially adjusted cars. With the new light weight collapsible wheel chairs, its owner is able to maneuver it into the car single handed. Sometimes this measure of independence is not enough. Society has been developed to mainly consider the needs of the able-bodied. This means that in some areas little consideration has been given to the needs of those less fortunate. The "Year of the Disabled" highlighted many of these shortcomings, particularly the need for ramps into buildings, disabled toilets and the designing of kitchens and home construction to be more friendly for the less agile of limb.

It may seem ironic that a person may be able to drive a car yet be unable to keep some appointments or go some place because of the building and the way it is constructed. They are frequently unfriendly to the physically impaired. Assistance to enable them to keep such appointments is an offer welcomed and appreciated.

One of the most helpful things a pastoral person can do is, where appropriate, to promote a spirit of independence as much as possible.

There may be jobs around the home such as changing tap washers or light bulbs, taking down or putting up curtains after washing, the heavier spring cleaning cannot be done by the handicapped unaided. Such assistance may be seen as pastoral care. The offer of such help should remain open and without embarrassment.

How can such be done without embarrassment?

Let the impaired see you as a buddy or companion. In other words they need to perceive you as an equal and as a good friend. Without that sense of being on the same level you may be seen as a patronizing "do-gooder". Such does not reflect the spirit of Christ or His Church.

In developing such a relationship of oneness, there is a freedom to ask for help without any sense of obligation or discomfort by a feeling of imposing on a friendship. Embarrassment has been thrown out the door and a relationship of true openness and friendship has been established in the spirit of Christ. When this happens both experience a giving and receiving of blessing though the relationship.

Facing intellectual and Theological Issues

Frustration, inadequacy, inferiority, hindrance, uncertainty, injustice are some of the confused feelings felt by the disabled, particularly in the early months of their disability and when they have time to consider what has happened. Hows, whys, what ifs and where are questions that fill and clog the mind.

The pastoral care person may be hit with such questions which are largely intellectual and theological. The theological ones may be filed away until they have tested and proved the genuineness of your care and interest in them, or they may be hurled bluntly and accusingly at you because of their anger at God over what has occurred.

How do you answer such questions as; how did this happen to me? What have I done to deserve this? What if I hadn't gone there? I can't think of any reason why I have been inflicted with this condition. These intellectual ponderings should be answered on that level. If you start to apply spiritual answers with responses like: God is in control, perhaps you did something that displeased God, God has a reason for it or did you bring it on yourself? To imply some judgment on them or that God is somehow involved is to disregard the possibility that they are very hostile toward God and no logical deduction for them is possible. To give cause to stir or further aggravate their anger may well raise irremovable barriers between you and them. You may be seen as being in league with the enemy.

Once intellectual issues have been worked through and sufficient confidence has been built up in you, it then may be time to tackle some of the theological queries. In any discussion, it should stress that God does not deliberately harm or hurt one of his creatures. The Psalmist in Psalm 121 asks the question, *"Will I look to the hills for help which are covered in shrines to man-made gods?"* He responds with a resounding, *"No! My help will come from the living God who made all things."* (*my personal paraphrase of Psalm 121 verses 1-2*)

That is the point to which theological questions should lead. The move to this point should be made very slowly and sensitively taken. You may not be able to reach that point, for some time if ever, because of bitterness and resentment against God. You are not a failure if you cannot deal with theological issues under such circumstances.

The presentation of theological issues must be seen to be associated with other aspects of practical care and concern, otherwise all such expositions may be considered as insincere and that the religious drive is seen to overrule genuine pastoral care to the whole person. Always the persons emotional and reasoning state should determine how far a conversation should proceed.

Long Term Interest and Care

Almost all incidents of impairment are life long sentences. The offering of pastoral car should not be confined to the acute period of the onset of the condition. Any ministry providing support for the disabled should be an ongoing commitment unless an amicable other suitable support network is able to be made.

The uncertainty and concern over how they will be able to manage their handicap fills them with apprehension and fear. They are fragile and their lives are unstable; they need stability and dependability around them. If they cannot rely on consistent pastoral care and interest, then, depression is one of the other alternatives which take over their mind and spirit. That support needs to be regular and not haphazard to suit the convenience of the carer. For the patient to feel that they are some sort of appendage to other interests and are not worthy of any deeper interest is denigrating and further humiliating for the patient. This can further dispirit the person causing a poor response to rehabilitation therapy.

Pastoral ministry to the disabled is demanding on time, energy and Christian grace.

Creating Opportunities

It is so easy for an impaired person to have feelings of being an isolated island and cut off from the mainstream of life. They cannot do or participate in many things that a strong able-bodied person is able to be involved in. They are constantly the spectator looking on as many of the pleasures and thrills of life pass them by.

What can a pastoral person do to relieve that sense of isolation and of being an encumbrance on the scene? Just to read the bible, pray or sermonize with them is likely to further alienate them. The carer must be proactive in assisting in introducing them to supportive specialist networking groups, other support groups and the church community.

Having facilitated support groups for leukemia patients, bereaved parents, and foster parents, an appreciation of the value of such groups is known.   The value of such groups is that they realize that they are not isolated lone rangers. There are other people like them, with the same problems which a few have overcome, such a support group gives them a sense of companionship with others who have or are still passing through the same waters. The encouragement from these experiences gives them the opportunity to see a light shining ahead along their dark road. Alcoholics Anonymous is a typical example of the value of such groups.

Efforts to be aware of such organizations should be one of the first tasks of a carer who begins to visit a handicapped person.

It is important that the patient knows of and has the opportunity to join such groups. A Hospital Social Work Department may provide the necessary information. Because they are not necessarily a Christian support group should not deter the person from belonging to the group. A conservative Christian background may make the disabled cautious about joining a non-church group. The carer should try to assist her to see the value of meeting people traveling along a similar road.

One of the carer's main tasks is to try to encourage integration back into social activity with other people. If it is a truly caring church, then the church is an ideal place to provide the needed understanding fellowship. Most churches have members who are shut-ins. They may not be able to sit for long during a church service or they may have urinary tract problems or other socially disabling condition. An informal getting together of such people who have to urgently go to the toilet or have to stand up every five minutes or so may be an alternative to attending a normal church service. It may be a purely social group, a bible study or special interest group or a mixture of these or other activities. If it meets the need for socialization and fellowship with some spiritual input it is filling an important need in the life of the handicapped. These groups build bridges between the isolation of incapacity and the mainstream of understanding, incorporation, fellowship and companionship.

A Rich Full Life

Disabled persons live in two worlds, the world of the handicapped and the world at large. The first can be embittering, hardening, unresponsive and self-centered. The second can be condescending, pitying, and self-centered. These pictures can promote in the one, 'what is the use of living?' Or in the whole bodied person 'by the grace of God there go I.' It could be seen as east and west and the never shall they meet. For many in both groups, that is their experience of or attitude to life. That is not the purpose or intention of God for mankind. God's intention or purpose is that we should live a rich and full life.

It has been my privilege to minister to and work with disabled people. A physical impairment does not necessarily mean that a fruitful life cannot be enjoyed. A delightful story appeared recently concerning a thirteen year old cerebral palsied girl who has aspirations to win a place in the national Olympic team for the 2008 Para Olympics in Beijing. A few weeks earlier it was mentioned that her parents required $10,000 to prepare for and send her to the games.

A man who was a Professor for thirty years at the Queensland University gave her parents a check for the full amount. This Professor has cerebral palsy. Both his and the girl's impairment were obvious on the television interviews. Is there any person in the world who had such a rewarding, rich and satisfying life than the severely handicapped physicist, Stephan Hawkins? He was one of the most brilliant minds of the last 100 years, whose contribution to the world of science has few equals.

Pastoral carers and the church should not look upon the disabled as second class citizens but as people with potential for leading full and satisfying lives within their limitations and be an inspiration to all they contact. The Church's role is to provide opportunities for the impaired to look and move forward rather than let them constantly reflect upon what they have lost. They should be encouraged to participate in church activities as far as they are able, inciting them to contribute to the extent of their restrictions. The showing of such confidence in them may have more effect than cough syrup to a sore throat.

Where these opportunities and facilities are not available at present in the church program, the Board, prompted by the Pastoral Committee, should seek out ways through which the numbers of disabled in the community may participate. Many are unchurched for the lack of the church's interest.

The church must remember that the impaired are very discerning of what the church is doing or not doing in pastorally caring for them.

CHAPTER 10

Coronary

Concerns

In the Western World, more people die of Cardiovascular Disease than any other, irrespective of ethnic roots. Many authorities in the United States report that just less than one million die each year from some form of heart disease. This represents 42% of all deaths.[15] From Canberra, Australia come similar reports with 39% of all deaths being due to cardiovascular disease. The number of heart failure deaths is 1.7 times greater amongst women over fifty years, as women usually start to develop coronary heart disease ten to fifteen years later than men.[16]

What is Cardiovascular Disease?

Cardiovascular disease, as the name suggests concerns the cardio (heart) and vascular (blood) vessels. It includes all those many illnesses that involve the smooth functioning of the heart and or blood vessels. The heart pumps 70 to 100 mls of blood around the body seventy times a minute, 100,000 times a day and two and a half million times in a life time. The heart pumps the blood through the arteries and capillaries to every part of the body and then back into the lungs where it is

---

[15] National Centre for Health Statistics, National; Centre for Chronic Disease Prevention and Health Promotion and Centre for Disease Control and Prevention. 1995.
[16] Australia Facts 2001. Australian Institute of Health and Welfare CUD NO.13.

reoxygenated with the recycled blood passing back into the heart.[17] Heart disease is caused by abnormal conditions which affect the quality of the blood, its flow and the function of the heart and the distribution by the blood vessels

As blood vessels supply fresh blood and remove the spent blood from all parts of the body they are the source of the supply of oxygen to vital parts such as heart, brain and other organs. If any of these parts are starved of oxygen and cleansed blood via the heart, through blockages or insufficient flow of blood, then the organ will slowly deteriorate or will suddenly stop. If the blockage is complete then a cardiovascular accident occurs.

Types of Cardiovascular Disease

Many conditions of heart disease are caused by or accelerated by unhealthy life styles. The risk of heart disease may be minimized or slowed by exercise, reduction of cholesterol levels, and carefully following an approved nutritional diet. Smoking has serious detrimental effects upon the cardiovascular system.

Not all heart conditions are due to life style. Cardiomyopathy may develop as a result of various viral attacks. Genetics and congenital defects are responsible for some cardiac problems. Severe mental stress or heart muscular strain through the wrong type of physical exertion, may also damage the heart. Twenty five years ago, I developed a heart condition which slowed and incapacitated me for normal work. It took months of tests and trials to establish that it was caused by an excessive consumption of caffeine, through strong hospital coffee which produced regular heart muscular spasm, causing irregular flow of the blood around the body with felt consequences. By eliminating caffeine intake for a period and now restricting myself to two cups of coffee per day, I have a normal, functioning, healthy cardiovascular system.

---

[17] Victor Chang Cardiac Research Institute, Sydney, Newsletter 27th April 2005.

Coronary Artery Disease (CAD)

These are diseases that are commonly known as heart attacks and are the result of a condition known as ***atherosclerosis.*** Starting in early childhood, the smooth inner-lining of the heart and blood vessels begin to clog up with material known as atherosclerotic plaque or simply plaque such as fat and cholesterol. This is also known as blocked arteries or narrowing of the arteries. This build up of plaque reduces the amount of oxygen and nutrients getting to the heart muscles. When this imbalance of supply and need for oxygen lasts for more than a few minutes it causes chest pressure or pain known as ***angina pectoris.*** Other symptoms may be heart burn, nausea, vomiting and heavy sweating. Repeated incidents can cause the heart muscle to die causing heart attacks and is known as a ***myocardial infarction. Arrhythmias or dysrhythmias and*** are also caused by the lack of blood flow that in many cases may also be a cause of sudden death.

Coronary artery disease is a disease of the arteries supplying the lungs only.

Heart Disease

Coronary Heart disease is the most common heart disease affecting the blood vessels. The term coronary heart disease is much broader than coronary artery disease in that it refers to the resultant complications of coronary artery disease. Heart impairment develops as a result of damage to either heart muscle tissue, the valves of the heart, or the development of disease within the vessels circulating the blood through the body. Forms of heart disease include:

- **Cardiomyopathy.** Cardiomyopathy occurs as the result of damage to heart muscles following a heart attack or other causes. Scar tissue often results from a heart attack damaging the muscle. Muscle damage affects the pumping efficiency of the heart. The heart's ability to contract while pumping becomes abnormal (***Systolic dysfunction)*** and the relaxing stage during the filling of the heart also may become damaged *(diastolic dysfunction).*

- **Valvular Heart Disease.** Inside the heart itself there are a number of valves connecting the various chambers which regulate the flow of blood in its rhythmic cycle. Valvular disease indicates that the normal blood flow from chamber to chamber is faulty because the valves are not shutting the blood off completely causing a leak when it contracts. This is known as *valvular regurgitation or valvular inefficiency.* A diseased valve may noticeably obstruct the blood flow known as *valvular stenosis.* A neonate may be born with valvular malformations which may require urgent corrective surgery. Damage can be done to the valves of the heart by viral or bacterial infections resulting in what is called **infectious endocarditis.**

- **Pericardial Disease.** Around the heart is a sac known as the pericardium. The pericardium may become inflamed, known as *pericarditis.* It may become filled with fluid *(pericardial efffusion)* or become stiff, causing *constrictive pericarditis.* Naturally each of these conditions affects the heart's efficiency

- **Congenital Disorders.** These may be detected at birth or sometime later. One or other of the various parts of the heart (its muscles, chambers, septa or valves) may be defective or a narrowed aorta may be restricting blood flow. Often, it is the malformation of the heart valves or the major heart vessels. When there is a hole between two heart chambers it is known as a hole in the heart. Surgery as soon after birth is necessary to correct many of these conditions and to allow the infant the opportunity of a normal healthy development through life.

- **Congestive Heart Failure.** This is the consequences of a dysfunction in the rhythmic functioning of the heart. Often organs which depend upon the regular supply of blood are inhibited in their function. Oxygen starved lungs will bring about shortness of breath and lung congestion. *Systolic (left sided) heart failure* occurs when insufficient blood is pumped into the circulatory system backing up leaked fluid into the lungs. *Diastolic (right sided) heart failure* happens when the stiffened muscles cannot fill up the chambers causing the fluid to build up in the ankles and legs. Often, fatigue and inability to sustain normal activity may be traced to congestive heart failure. The development of congestive heart failure is linked to coronary artery disease, cardiomyopathy, valvular heart disease, hypertension and congenital heart disease weakening and damaging the heart.

- **High Blood Pressure.** There is a high incidence of high blood pressure in the western world. The measurement of blood pressure is able to give some indication of the condition of the arteries. The more clogged with plaque they are, the narrower the arteries are to allow the blood to pass through. The higher the blood pressure, the harder the heart is pumping to supply the body with blood. The higher the blood pressure, the greater the risk of a cardiovascular attack. High blood pressure puts dangerous extra pressure on the artery walls which can cause them to rupture causing an internal hemorrhage. The increased pressure may cause some of the plaque to flake off sending it further along the artery until it reaches a narrower restriction of the vessel causing a complete blockage. Strokes occur in this way by blocking the flow of blood to the brain. High blood pressure is known to affect the kidneys and the eyes as well as predisposing to coronary heart disease and congestive heart failure.

- **Aneurysm.** Imagine a bicycle tire tube which has a weak spot in its wall? If you continue to increase the air pressure it will balloon out at that weak point with the balloon wall being very thin and fragile. It can easily burst causing all the air to escape. An aneurysm is the ballooning out of such a weak spot on an artery wall. When it bursts it empties the blood into the surrounding body cavity. A burst aneurysm in most cases is quickly fatal. When diagnosed, surgery is immediately ordered to repair the aneurysm and prevent it rupturing and avoid a hemorrhage. In most cases, the weakness in the artery's wall has been there since prebirth and has in fact been like a time bomb ready to explode at any time. Cerebral aneurysms are almost certainly congenital. Men, in early adulthood to pre middle years, without warning, may have such a fatal accident without warning. ***Aortic aneurysm*** is an aneurysm which occurs in the wall of the main artery, the aorta, leading from the heart itself. Should it burst, it fills the abdominal capacity with the uncontrollable escaping blood. If it bursts, it is fatal. The risk remains high even for a patient who has been diagnosed with an aortic aneurism and is rushed into the operating theater for repair

- **Thrombosis.** A thrombosis is a clot in a blood vessel. There are two types of thrombosis – **venous and arterial**. A thrombosis obstructs the flow of blood through the circulatory system. Venous thrombosis mostly occurs in the leg either in the superficial veins or in the deep veins. A **superficial venous thrombosis** causes discomfort without serious damage and remains in the place where it formed. The **deep venous thrombosis** is usually found in the deep veins of the leg or pelvic area. It blocks the vein causing pain and swelling behind the blockage and a burning redness around the swollen area. Such a clot may break up and start to move, frequently lodging in the lungs causing a **pulmonary embolism**. This type of floating clot, between the heart and the brain, can cause a stroke due to the restriction of oxygen to the brain by the reduction in the blood flow.

- When medium or large sized arteries thicken, it is known as **atherosclerosis.** They account for a large percentage of heart attacks. When the coronary arteries are affected, it causes a reduction in the blood supply to the heart muscles. Atherosclerosis may develop into **arterial thrombosis** which commonly occurs in the coronary arteries, carotid or vertebral arteries, renal or placental arteries. Venous thrombosis, along with atherosclerosis and varicose veins, are varieties of peripheral vascular disease as they are often a distance from the heart chamber itself.

- **Palpitations.** These are extra heart beats or premature ventricular contractions. This is an indication of some irritation of the lower part of the heart's pumping system. The normal beat is noticeably affected. Palpitations can cause dizziness or shortness of breath. They can occur when there is severe anxiety, or a sudden shock or fright or a thyroid condition. There are other factors such as over ingestion of caffeinated products and alcohol. Another, not so common, condition predisposing to palpitations is just before menopause or other changing hormone levels. These are usually harmless.

- **Arrhythmias.** Similar to palpitations are arrhythmias which are identified as missed heart beats, increased heart beats or an unusual fluttering in the chest. The occasional dizzy spell, shortness of breath, vague chest pain or faintness may be due to arrhythmia. Often the person is alarmed by such new experiences or their frequent occurrence. To relieve any building up of anxiety, they should be encouraged to see their doctor.

The Mind and Heart Disease

Both before and after the diagnosis of heart disease, the mind continues to have an influential role. There are many factors which may be involved in the development of heart disease. We have already seen the various types of cardiac illnesses and have become aware that they are not all from the same origin but may have various causes. One area in which knowledge is incomplete is the relation between stress and the onset of heart disease in some people.

Stress and Cardiovascular Disease
Most in the medical profession agree that there is a linkage between the two. Stress is considered to be a contributing factor in high blood pressure. Stress may also be a serious secondary contribution to heart function deterioration. Many stressed people turn to smoking, alcohol, binge eating, poker machines, or an addiction to take-away fatty foods which raise cholesterol levels or they may seek consolation in promiscuous sex, all of which will create more problems and further anxiety. Whether stress was involved or not in producing the original heart or other cardiovascular condition, these new methods to escape the stress of the diagnosis may have more serious damaging repercussions on the cardiovascular system.
Stress is blamed for some of our moods and reactions. Stress over illness is due to the pressures and claims of our family, social and employment responsibilities that may be threatened. Some will say that they are taking things in their stride. To admit to being under stress is another way of declaring that there is a problem, whether it is emotional, physical or financial and that you are not coping. Therefore we cannot deny the fact that we are stressed to a greater or lesser degree from time to time. Where the heart is already weak and the stress increases, the heart maybe damaged, blood pressure will build up with little relief.

The effect of stress upon the function of the Cardio-vascular system will depend upon the amount of time spent on brooding over the negative implications of the problem(s) while ignoring positive remedies and moving to implement these.

Experts in stress management suggest diet, exercise, group work and relaxation techniques for stress relief. These can be helpful, but insufficient as they offer some short term relief so long as the regimen is strictly adhered to. The root cause or causes of the stress may not be dealt with. There is a need to understand the real cause of the stress and deal with it. If it is financial, help is needed to understand budgeting and a better way to manage the financial situation. Emotional stress in relationships, marriage, family, and workplace may need the advice of a special counselor or a decision to spend some time away from the problem to gain some perspective and make practical decisions. The less obvious stress generators are our own expectations, the need to impress others, to be respected and other behavioral patterns which can become disruptive of factors in our lives and antagonistic to others.

Emotional and Psychological Changes after a Heart Event.
A cardiovascular event brings necessary changes to the life of the patient. These provide challenges. Challenges of any sort create emotional and psychological stress. In order to master the challenge, a cardiac patient has to learn to manage chest pain in order to minimize the possibility of another attack. In doing so, certain previously enjoyable activities or other more strenuous outdoor pleasures have to be curtailed. All of a sudden future plans have to be discarded or seriously modified and others put on hold until necessary life style changes are known and accepted. Studies show that up to 25% of patients remain depressed for up to twelve months, up to 27% experience sub-clinical depression and 45% of these progress onto clinical depression. Other psychological effects include anger, aggressiveness, intolerance and hostility. Up to 25% of cardiac patients develop deep anxiety which leads to panic disorder. Any twinge of chest pain sends them into a panic, assuming that it is the end. This creates added anxiety and impatience which is reflected in the family's growing alarm over such actions. Up to 25% of marriages report a loss of communication and intimacy. These increasing tensions cause the spouses to become more stressed, exacerbating the deterioration of the relationship.[18]

When a depressed heart patient indicates that they are not willing or ready to accept or adapt to the changes necessary to their lifestyle, they are known to have 34% lower adherence rate to medical programs,

---

[18] Januzzi J.L., Stern T., Pastenak R.C, et al/ *The influence of anxiety and depression on outcome of patients with coronary artery disease.* Archives of Internal Medicine 2000; 160: 913-1921.

dietary regimens, smoking bans and self discipline in social situations e.g. physical exertion, eating etc. However, when depressed cardiac sufferers are encouraged and respond to a restoration of self-esteem and social acceptability, this increases their ability to make the changes in their lives that will promote improved health and a happier outlook on life.

In a paper, Guck, Kavan, Elsasser and Barone of Creighton University School of Medicine, Omaha, Nebraska suggest that up to 65% of patients with acute myocardial problems experience depression with 15% to 20% developing major depression. They have a 3.5 times higher risk of mortality than other CVD patients. They recommend cognitive-behavioral therapy that will help the patients to deal with environment, thoughts, emotions, behavior and physiology.[19]

Pastoral Intervention

The pastoral visitor to a heart patient even with some understanding of the foregoing will appreciate that in entering into a heart patient's personal life he or she may encounter a diversity of emotional attitudes. As research has shown, the majority of heart patients develop some sort of depression, whether it is mild or a major depressive state. The average pastoral visitor is not qualified or experienced enough to get seriously involved with serious depression. It often requires psychotherapy, including cognitive therapy, some knowledge of the pharmacology of the medication being taken as well as a medical awareness of the twists and turns of cardiac disease and reactions to treatment for it. Because a person has known or lived with a person who has had a similar condition still does not qualify them to know how the current patient feels, will not feel, function or will not function. Each case is different and requires professional expertise.

There are aspects of heart disease which can cause different reactions from those of cancer patients and disabled people. Many of the responses may be similar anger, grief, guilt regret, frustration and so on. Many people, particularly women, experience a cardiovascular event over the age of sixty. The effect of the illness then is not only borne by

---

[19] American Family Physician: 2001; 64:641-8, 651-2.

the patient, it is acutely felt in the lives of the family members, friends and close associates who may also be filled with fears, questions, guilt, regrets and anger over the threatened loss of the much loved heart patient. They may feel that problems in their past relationship need to be resolved before it is too late or doubts over how they will manage without their loved one and friend. Illness within a family or relationship creates tensions. The familiar pattern of life changes or is threatened. The seriousness of the threat will only be realized as each person's reaction to the illness becomes evident, though family members may recognize the need to bond together to meet the crisis, it is always not possible. Personalities differ, and for some the care and nurturing is too much, and the result is separation and loneliness. If too much love and concern is shown, perhaps this will make the parting even more difficult. So anticipatory grief takes over and emotional ties are loosened. The onset of a cardiac attack in some cases is the beginning of the end of the family unit as a whole and precipitates the loss of some of the family's closeness.

With other families, the crisis has a more positive effect. The health crisis of the family member encourages each member of the family to take stock: hurts, slights, injustices, insensitivities, and taking each other for granted. These should have been openly confronted ten, twenty or thirty years earlier and only now begin to be faced by confession, forgiveness and healing that bring each closer to the other.. A fresh, deeper and more intimate relationship unites and strengthens the family.

As no two patients experience their heart attack in the same way or under similar conditions so all families will not deal or cope with the crisis in the same way. All families and spouses face a change in the needs and demands of its members specially the one who is ill. The spouse of the heart patient may have been dependent upon the patient for financial, emotional or physical support for their own infirmity.

The pastoral visitor may find himself or herself in families in differing stages of family reintegration or disintegration due to the illness. Early awareness of the family dynamics is essential if a useful pastoral relationship is to be established. Where there is disintegration, the reception may be cool. The family or some of them may see the visitor as intruding into a very personal situation. If there is anger with God over the illness, a visitor with a strong faith may not be welcome. In such a situation the visitor should avoid comment, other than concern and care and concentrate on the patient, providing as much emotional support and solace as possible. Be aware that the patient may be feeling guilty because he or she has ignored previous medical warnings. While the family is coming to grips with their own tensions, angers, fears and frustrations, any religious applications at that stage by the visitor are unlikely to be helpful. The emotional states of the patient and the family must be the carer's priority before deeper spiritual issues are discussed.

Awareness of the Patient's Feelings

There are a number of emotional states that may develop with the onset of heart disease. Even after successful bypass surgery, these may well have a bearing not only on the patient but also on the family and associates.

- Preoccupation with the fear of death. When will the next attack occur?
- Doubts over future ability to return to normal activities or adjust to the physical impairment. Will I always be an invalid?
- Facing the normal questions in crisis. Why? How can I? Why Now? What will happen to ...?
- Dependant on a medical environment of tests, more test, medication and uniforms. What will they tell me next?
- The effect of medication on their mind, perception and physical resources. Will I ever be able to think straight again?
- Dependence upon others and being out of control of their own body. What will the Doctor do to me next?

The pastoral visitor should recognize that most of these are negative responses to their condition and are beyond his or her expertise to make a substantial difference except to encourage the patient in whatever rehabilitation is prescribed. It needs to be reinforced that they should not be too despondent if the progress is slow or is taking longer than they thought. The visitor should try to:

i. Encourage the patient to take up new interests and activities within their restricted abilities e.g. crosswords, jigsaw puzzles, scrapbooking, board games with others.

ii. Encourage the patient to view the change of circumstances as a challenge and to see and live life from a different aspect. Whatever the circumstances, negatives can be made less hurtful by a positive outlook and attitude. All is not lost while there is breath and an active mind.

iii. Enable them to see that openness and expression of feelings with family members will break down communication barriers many of which may have been there for decades.

   a. Stress the value of finalizing all unfinished business even if it includes confessing some earlier shameful or embarrassing life Interventions. In matters affecting spouse and family, these should be confessed, rectified and forgiven no matter who is to blame or the seriousness of the episodes.

To raise any of these issues, a good rapport with the patient and family must first be established with a willingness to quickly drop any such initiative if the reception brings out frosty or negative responses. If accepted, then there will be benefits in attitude, peace of mind and importantly, in the patient's attitude to the medical condition. With the relieving of such stressors, a happier and more cooperative atmosphere will be enjoyed.

The patient will feel he or she is included fully within the family. Family plans and discussions will be trusting and open. A deeper sense of love and intimacy in personal sharing may be expected. Husband and wife will be able to anticipate with eagerness their sharing of love and those more meaningful moments of passion that seemed to have become forbidden territory since the fall out from the cardiovascular attack.

The Carer and the Spiritual Dimension

If your ministry has been able to touch any of these areas with the patient or family members, it has had a spiritual dimension. Spiritual healing has taken place in one or more hearts. Here, we should note that spiritual verses, religious ministration, religious formulas involves or invokes specific religious aspects associated with the formulas, rites or the background of those involved. A family stricken with a loved one with heart disease may find it difficult to think of faith or religion in those terms when in their minds they are questioning. How can a loving, caring God allow this to happen to me or us? To hear pious religious turns of phrase when their minds are so confused and antagonistic creates added tension. The other question which may also plague the mind is the inevitable guilt laden one. What have I done to deserve this?

One proposes an indifferent God; the second implies a wrathful judgmental God. Both of these concepts have the reverse effect upon the healing potential of the human body. Guilt ingrains self-condemnation; judgmental anger inflicts hopelessness. It is the spirituality, including a religious perceptiveness, that is without any sense of sermonizing or evangelical fervor that is able to sit quietly alongside the patient and those concerned with the patient and listen to where they are at, as they grapple with these questions.

One must be continually aware of the deeply religious person who will hang on every word or scripture offered. However, care must be taken not to use their religious background to build false and unrealistic hopes for the patient. Often such patients expect to be the recipients of a Divine miracle.

The patient and family are also grappling with the grief that the illness has thrust upon them. The pastoral visitor must be conscious of the delicacy of such a hurtful situation that the family is passing through. To say the wrong thing adds further turmoil into the situation. The right approach is able to bring relief, peace, hope and the restoration of faith. It is a very responsible position in which to be placed that can only be accepted and fulfilled with the help of God's wisdom, presence and patience.

It must be reiterated; the God most people acknowledge whether Christian or otherwise is compassionate, loving and merciful. Therefore the patient needs to realize:

- Whatever the cause, nobody deserves heart disease.
- It has happened and the occurrence cannot be denied or eliminated although in some cases it may be healed, eased or made bearable.
- A positive outcome can be achieved by making the patient and family members more aware of the value of life and make their lives more sensitive, caring and empathetic toward others. This will help to minimize the personal bitterness over the illness.
- Anger, whether it be toward the illness, their own foolishness and carelessness, family members, medical staff or God, is unjust or unwarranted. Anger needs to be expressed. Direct it toward the condition, itself. The anger can be expressed by physical exertion such as with a piece of hose, wood or a pillow against a post, the mattress or other non-destructible object. I had the hospital authorities attach padded panels to the walls in the emergency room and intensive care relatives' waiting rooms. These saved frequent repairs to broken walls from irate relative's fists.

Wrongly placed anger has negative repercussions:

- ❖ Against ourselves. It depresses
- ❖ Against others. It alienates.
- ❖ Against God. It destroys faith and rejects the spiritual support of God and religion.

Conversely, physically expressed anger relieves the depressing effects of the confusion and mental turmoil that has been built up and it releases much of the tension allowing the mind to think more clearly.

- There is need to concentrate on what they have instead of what has been negatively affected.
- Attitude to the future must be to make the most of their lives sharing love and encouragement with those around them in a spirit of gratitude and thanksgiving for past blessings, anticipating the continuing presence and watchfulness of God over them.
- Anticipate strength, peace and blessing from previously un-encountered sources.
- Seek out and foster fellowship and relationships with people who will provide a continuing, growing stability in their spiritual lives.
- Where permission has been given and appropriate, prayer is able to sustain, and give strength to cope with the pain and the anxiety of watching over the loved one incapacitated and the stress of the one ill.

The pastoral person, by the right cooperation with God, may be able to turn the physical disaster of heart disease into true spiritual growth of a close personal relationship with God for all concerned. This objective will not always be completed in part or in whole. Whatever doors begin to open in dealing with a heart disease patient and the family, only a gentle entry with genuine, empathetic, sensitivity is able to start to reach this goal. Whatever the result at the end, to be able to say that you walked with God into that family's crisis, were a companion to them in their trials, offered what they were able to accept at that time and did not over stretch the boundaries of the encounter, will bring its own reward.

CHAPTER 11
Spirituality
And
Well-Being

A whole human being must be integrated in body, mind and spirit. This integration is the determining factor in human composure. If anyone of these states is in poor health it will have its effect upon the other elements. Thus an infection or organic illness in a person's body will affect the person's mental attitude and thus in turn affects the ability of the spirit to generate and project the enthusiasm needed to maintain harmony within the person and with the world about him. Thus, inner peace, love, strength, and serenity are in danger of impairment.

When the mind is in turmoil, troubled or ill at ease, psychosomatic illnesses and illnesses of the spirit are likely to appear. Likewise, when the spirit is crippled and unable to attain its normal serenity and divine communication, it is unable to pacify the mind or stimulate the body to positive responses.

The importance of this integration is becoming more widely recognized and accepted. The development of the disciplines of psychology and psychiatry has identified the relationship between the body and the mind. It is only in the last fifty years, that the spiritual aspect of man has become significant for its relationship to the other two members of this human trinity. Unfortunately, its importance has been lessened when given a religious label. That is what Peach called it. [20] He wrote that religion is a powerful factor influencing health, well-being and medical decisions for better or for worse and that a patient's faith should not be ignored or neglected by physicians. Peach, here, as well as others, who have written on the subject, medical or otherwise, are less than exact when they call it religion. The correct terminology is spirituality. Religion involves adherence to a certain set of rules and dogmas of a structured institution dedicated to the worship and devotion of a particular deity or deities. Often it is merely a mental assent to what has been taught, with little involvement of the spirit.

Spirituality in these last fifty years has become better understood as interfaith and ecumenical openness has brought about an acceptance that there is more than one way of communicating with and experiencing the reality of spiritual powers beyond our world. With this deeper spiritual awareness we recognize that most religious traditions acknowledge the connection between spirituality and health. From earliest times, primal religion was concerned with placating spirits to restore health.

Spirituality has been defined in many ways. It is claimed to be the way a person finds meaning, hope, comfort and inner peace in life. Many would tell us that they find the presence of God through the observance of religious ritual which is intended to focus upon and enhance a consciousness of the presence of God. Many Christians, for example, maintain their spirituality through regular meaningful participation in the Eucharist. Others in the same service may experience little because it is purely a formal religious practice. Their spirit has not been engaged in the rite. Others may find their own daily scripture reading and prayer, involvement in music, art, reflection on nature are ways by which their spirit reaches out to their source of spiritual inspiration.

---

[20] Peach, H.G. Religion Spirituality and Health: How should Australia's medical professions respond? Med. J. Aust 2003; 178: 86-88

This differs from bodily health, which refers to the state of the organic physical body. Mental health incorporates feelings and attitudes of well-being. Spiritual health deals with values and meanings. If a person's values are focused upon the material things, then, greed, selfishness and self aggrandizement may become significant, which is a sign of poor spiritual health. Yet such persons might be very religious, regularly attending all the accepted rituals. The drive for wealth and power may become obsessive, which destroys the body's balance and its capacity to deal with pressures created by this obsession, resulting in burn-out and a breakdown in health... A healthy person with spiritual values sees the advantages in working for peace and harmony within themselves, others, and in the natural environment.

Adrian Lyons[21] brings out thoughts on spirituality into a modern context when he sees spirituality as being related to a prayer tradition from a respected teacher. It may also be attained through meditation. There are various types of meditation using mantras, yoga and contemplation or a set of routine exercises such as Tai Chi or even receiving encouragement and inspiration from memories of deceased loved ones. Simply put, a person may become consciously aware of his or her spirituality through paths that are familiar to a cultural tradition or that have been uncovered through sincere personal search. Lyons says, "The element common to spiritualities is receptiveness linked to a conviction that someone or something, beyond one's physical senses, provides valuable guidance." He cites Patrick O'Sullivan's[22] definition of spirituality as "a way of living that feeds our spirit – which is our capacity to relate in a free and loving way with God and the rest of creation." When this supernatural source of our spirituality is the center of our thanksgiving, adoration and intercession, it is at its most meaningful and richest.

How does all this relate to our well-being? Our spirit needs to be healthy for the mind and body to function at its best. In earlier chapters we have seen the effects grief, depression, uncertainty, cancer, heart disease,

---

[21] Lyons Adrian. Imagine believing (David Lovell: Melbourne) 2003 pp. 79-80
[22] O'Sullivan Patrick. God knows how to come back home (Aurora Book: Melbourne) 1999, p.vii.

guilt, and disability, amongst many other things, have upon our body, mind and spirit. In many cases, the whole being may fall apart with these ills making it almost impossible for us to efficiently fulfill the demands of life. Each of these factors will bring about deterioration in the functioning of body, mind and spirit.

The pastoral person needs to be conscious of the interplay of these when making a pastoral visit. The spirit has a vital role to play in all matters and this should not be overlooked, taken for granted or minimized. The average pastoral carer has not the expertise or experience in medicine or psychiatry to directly and fully deal with those elements. However by encouraging some spiritual response the other two aspects of the patient may be improved.

Understanding the necessity for wholeness is the mark of a very observant, and compassionate pastoral helper. The danger, though, is in thinking that anyone can usefully impose any kind of spiritual formula or ritual upon another person, without that person's full acceptance and agreement.

By careful listening and sensitive responses, a thoughtful person may be able to ascertain the spiritual situation or status of the patient, but if this does not readily emerge, it should not be pressed. Until further discussion or changed circumstances give evidence of the patient's willingness to provide further insight into his spiritual state.

The spirit has a vital role to play in all matters and this should not be overlooked, taken for granted or minimized

Only when there is a sign of positive acceptance or some slight evidence of religious interest, you might cautiously say just before leaving. "Would you like me to pray with you now or some other time?" A negative response arouses no resentment and is easily brushed off with, "some other time." That of course, may mean 'never'. The reaction to such a request may or may not indicate that overt spiritual care is not desired from you. Depending upon the nature of the negative response your parting words may be, "I'll remember you in my prayers and may God bless you." This leaves the door open and confirms the sincerity of your intentions and interest.

Earlier it has also been suggested that the one being visited should be encouraged to focus upon the positives rather than the negatives in their situation and the importance of forgiveness etc. These address mental states, but they will also help remove the blockages to spiritual health. One of the least useful aspects of pastoral care which has emerged in recent years is the way in which some pastoral workers have taken on the role of pseudo-psychologists and pseudo-psychiatrists. The dangers inherent in this approach are obvious.

Such an attitude by those even with some clinical background may easily permit the psychological to outweigh the important spiritual values in the communication. For the pastoral worker, the spiritual should always be the critical and important factor. Leave the patient's other needs to the trained and accredited specialist.

A pastoral person is able to leave the medical and psychological in the hands of expert medical and qualified psychologists. Belief and spiritual experience have an important place alongside medicine and psychology in the restoration of the person to lasting wholeness.

A person should not take on regular pastoral visitation without some serious training in pastoral care. I would strongly suggest that such visitation should also include a serious strand of supervision of the pastoral visits by a qualified person or in the context of the pastoral care team. Any course or courses being sought should include supervision or praxis among other aspects of pastoral encounters in the hospital situation.

When Jesus sent his disciples into the villages they had to report back to him. Jesus supervised his disciples' pastoral ministry. Pastoral visitation through the church should be organized by a Pastoral Care Team to whom regular reports should be made. Ideally the team should participate in a regular monthly in-service training group It may prove that one person rather than another is more suitable for this particular ministry. Paul clearly stated in his letter to the Ephesians, chapter 4 that the Holy Spirit has given different gifts to each believer. It is well worthwhile to spend some time seeking to understand your true gift for ministry and not just choosing what you would like to do. Some of my students who have a high opinion of their skills I would not willingly let loose on pastoral visitation. Their demeanor is abrasive and condescending. Their personalities are not endearing and warm. These are things the pastoral care team should be quick to assess. Other avenues of ministry should be found for them but they should not be included in the team even if they have completed a course or three. Better to have one unhappy person than have many people alienated from the church and helpful spiritual resources, by one visitor's insensitivity, unfortunate personality or lack of pastoral perceptiveness. We would hope that the pastoral care team will develop and foster in the pastoral person a healthy spiritual outlook whose own spirituality is being cultivated and maintained by prayer and application.

A pastoral ministry's primary concern is the well-being of the whole person in body, mind and spirit. As the medical practitioner and the psychologist accept a high degree of responsibility in the discharge of their role so the pastoral carer must similarly understand his or her responsibility to provide the highest degree of proficient pastoral care through ministering to the spiritual needs of the person.

Every pastoral intervention requires sensitivity, and perceptivity. These are the hallmarks of pastoral care with the ill and dying.

Worship That Pleases God · by James W. Bartley, Jr. (PhD)
February 2008, 360 pages, 6' x 9'

ISBN 9780756884 (Paperback: US $17.99, UK £13.99) Category:
Non-fiction

James W. Bartley Jr. has gone beyond the common status quo to explore a subject that most authors do   not have sufficient experiential credentials to delve into. He practically reflects on his more than 60 years experience of walking with God to bring many into an awe-striking deeper communion with God.   His book, *Worship That Pleases God* gives an accurate insight into   the inexhaustible subject of Worship –   as an invaluable asset   in   the Man-God   relationship. Being a retired Professor   of theology, Dr. Bartley has successfully   made   a   holistic   and unassailable exposition of   worship –   as a theme that finds its root in   the book   of Genesis and continues to Revelation in   the Bible, while his   academic   perception   lends credence to   his work. Worship that pleases God is not just a book that enriches the knowledge of inquisitive readers; Dr. Bartley has carefully sequenced it in   such a manner that even the least motivated reader will simply find the wave of his discovered supernatural worship pattern so irresistible.

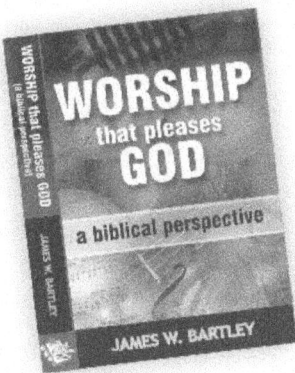

Order from www.baalhamon.com

The Fatherless – a novel by Erin Inman
February 2008, 420 pages, 5.5' x 8.5'
ISBN 9780756914 (Paperback: US $17.99, UK £13.99) Category: Fiction

Nick Pierce, a talented young boy whose singular obsession is music, finds himself overturned from a lonely life with his grandmother in Wichita, Kansas to the rather strange atmosphere of life in Western Kansas with the father he had never met. Although a friendly neighbor couple takes Nick under their wing, circumstances in life and his father's attitude work against him. In search for a way to fulfill his uttermost desires, he enters into a world of the unknown – a stranger world that leads him into questioning right from wrong. In the face of a life-threatening sickness, Nick wonders if life could offer him a little more, if music may still flow from his fingers, in praise to the Father-God.

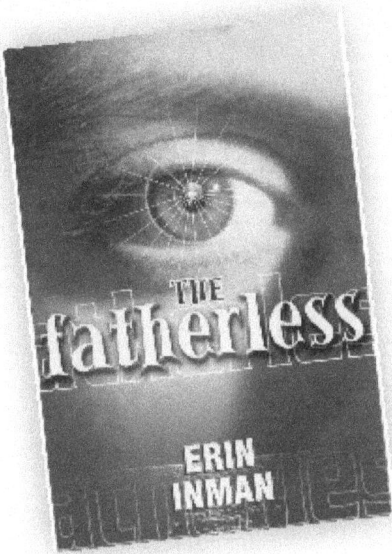

Also from Baal Hamon Publishers:

Take Me Home Windrider – by Jeff Knighton
July 2010, 264 pages, 5.5' x 8.5'
ISBN 9784956500 (Paperback: US $15.99) Category: Non-fiction

God uses nature to teach us His ways. God has taught Dr. Knighton to be a true Christian from his uniquely rich experience as a ranch hand in Texas. It was there that he enjoyed the tough but fulfilling labors of working with horses and cattle. The work offered plenty of hours under the deep Texan sky, in both kind and harsh weather, to examine his own spirit as he rode pasture observing nature, and tending to the cattle under his watch. This book captures the reflections that have given Dr. Knighton a perspective on life unique to those who have been privileged to spend time as a working cowboy which over the years has enhanced his work as a teacher and preacher. These reflections have been used as discussion starters in small group Bible studies, and as illustrations in preaching. They afford the reader an adventurous ride in the inner man with Christ.

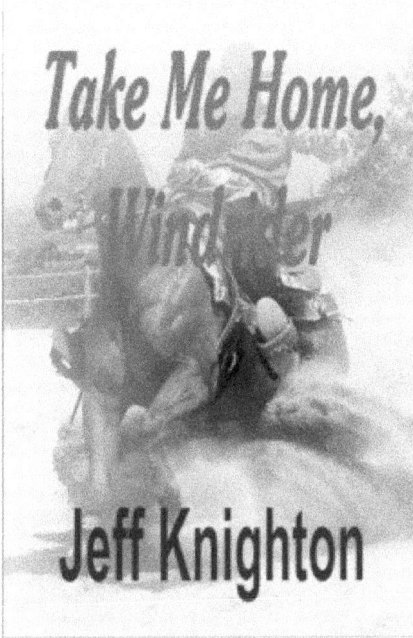

Order from www.baalhamon.com

Does God Truly Exist? – by Temitope Oyetomi
August 2006, 360 pages, 6' x 9'
ISBN 9780756825 (Paperback: US $17.99) Category: Non-fiction

Archbishop Akinola, Primate of the Church of Nigeria (Anglican Communion) 2000 – 2010, commends this book as a "valuable material for anyone tired of dodging the questions". Indeed, it is one book that has "*raised a fathom of questions*", as yet another Bishop - a PhD-holder - observes in the foreword. However, the tact with which the author resolves many of these questions is scholarly and engaging. The author writes with confidence and his arguments are intelligent and highly persuasive: facts and their interpretations are presented in a style that is approachable, digestible and amenable to reading by a wide audience. Ordinarily, one might think of it as a book for those who are in doubt of God's existence. Of course, it is. But it will be more applicable to those who are sure that God exists and who believe they are worshiping the true and living God. "*Who really is the true and living God*" and "*how best can one relate with God*" are the ultimate quests of the book.

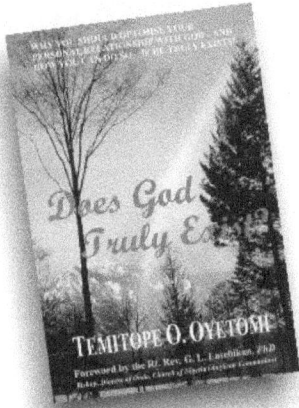

Drawing answers from science, religion and philosophy, the author has contrived a rare blend "*that will plausibly challenge every mind*". No wonder a Baptist minister recommends it "to all people no matter their religious persuasions". It is certainly an intellectual masterpiece.

www.ingramcontent.com/pod-product-compliance
Lightning Source LLC
Chambersburg PA
CBHW051952090426
42741CB00008B/1367